ART AND ESSENCE OF CANINE MASSAGE
PETMASSAGE™ FOR DOGS

Art and Essence of Canine Massage
PetMassage™ for Dogs

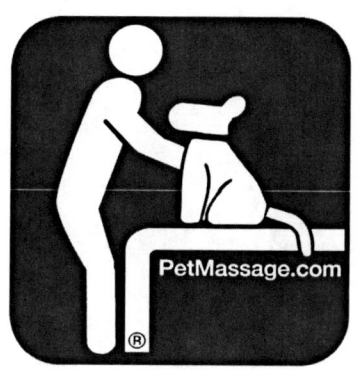

Art and Essence of Canine Massage

PetMassage™ for Dogs

ART AND ESSENCE OF CANINE MASSAGE
PETMASSAGE~TM~ FOR DOGS

ART AND ESSENCE OF CANINE MASSAGE
PETMASSAGE™ FOR DOGS

Art and Essence of Canine Massage

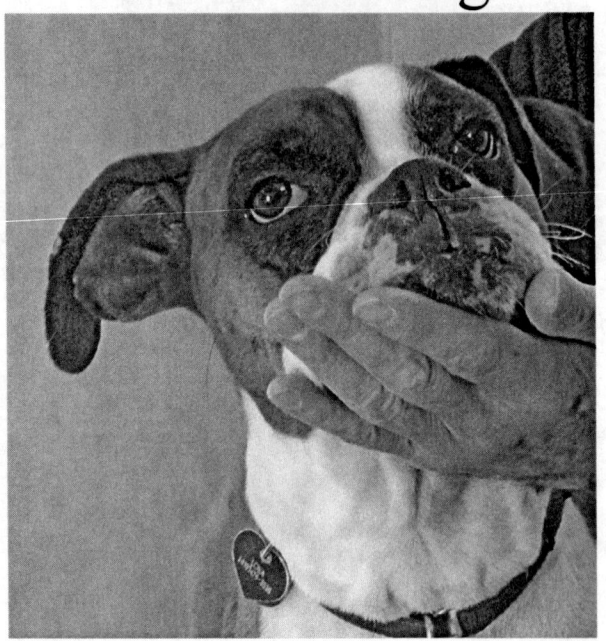

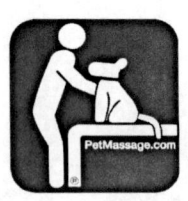

PetMassage™ for Dogs

Jonathan Rudinger

Founder and Director
PetMassage
Training and Research Institute

ART AND ESSENCE OF CANINE MASSAGE
PETMASSAGE™ FOR DOGS

ART AND ESSENCE OF CANINE MASSAGE
PETMASSAGE_{TM} FOR DOGS

Art and Essence of Canine Massage
PetMassage_{TM} for Dogs

Jonathan Rudinger

Includes bibliographical references
1. Pet Care   2. Dogs—Social Aspects—Anecdotes   3. Holistic Animal Care
4. Massage Dog PetMassage   5. Alternative Veterinary   6. Acupressure
7. Animal Communication 8. Dogs—Therapeutic—Anecdotes
9. Human Animal Relationships   10. PetMassage_{TM} Training & Research Institute

Cover Design Jonathan Rudinger
Photographs by Jonathan and Anastasia Rudinger

Art and Essence of Canine Massage PetMassage_{TM} for Dogs

Copyright © 2012 Jonathan Rudinger. *All rights reserved.*
Printed in the United States of America.
No part of this book may be reproduced or transmitted in any form or by any means, electronic or mechanical, including photocopying, recording, or by any information storage and retrieval system, without the permission in writing from the author.

For convenience and aesthetics in this book, the TM subscript has not been used after the word, "PetMassage." "PetMassage" is a Trademarked term. It has been owned and used solely by the PetMassage, Ltd and PetMassage Books, since 1998.

PetMassage_{TM} and its logo, the image of a person massaging a dog, on a rectangular background, are the Registered trademarks of
PetMassage_{TM}, Ltd., 3347 McGregor Lane, Toledo, OH 43623 USA.

For information contact PetMassage Books, PetMassage, Ltd.
3347 McGregor Lane, Toledo, OH 43623 USA.
www.PetMassage.com

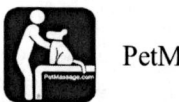 PetMassage_{TM} Books

PRINT EDITION

ISBN 978-0-9822102-7-7

ART AND ESSENCE OF CANINE MASSAGE
PETMASSAGE~TM~ FOR DOGS

Also by Jonathan Rudinger

Effective Pet Massage for Dogs, Manual

Effective Pet Massage for Dogs, DVD

Effective Pet Massage for Older Dogs, DVD

PetMassage for Dogs 1, DVD

PetMassage for Dogs 2, DVD

PetMassage for the Family Dog, Book

PetMassage: Energy Work With Dogs, Accessing The Magnificent Body Language and Body Wisdom of the Dog, Book and 5 Audio CD Set

Transitions, PetMassage Energy Work for the Aging and Dying Dog, Book

Creating & Marketing Your Animal Massage Business, Book

Dogs Kids PetMassage, Book

PetMassage: A Kid's Guide to Massaging Dogs, DVD

PetMassage: Doggie Songs for Kids, Audio CD

ART AND ESSENCE OF CANINE MASSAGE
PETMASSAGE™ FOR DOGS

PetMassage is the intentional touch of an animal's physical body for the purpose
of assisting him/her toward greater harmony and balance.

PetMassage enhances awareness to every part of the body
where it is touched.

Through the stimulation of myofascial referral zones
the areas of the animal's body not touched,
are affected as well.

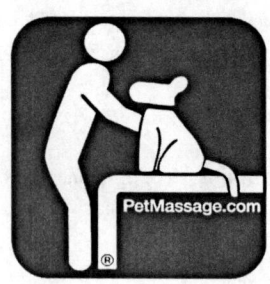

No one can see for another, not one.
No one can feel for another, not one.
No one can hear for another, not one.
No one can experience for another, not one.
No one can achieve for another, not one.
No one can grow for another, not one.
No one can live for another, not one.

However…

You can help another interpret what they see.
You can help another gain sensitivity in touch.
You can help another understand what they hear.
You can set the stage for experience.
You can help another make the most of what they have.
You can help create a climate for growth.
You can help make life more worth living.

      - Anonymous

With the active combination of skilled touch, compassion, and intention, PetMassage creates an ambient environment within the dog's body, mind and spirit.

An ambient environment
is necessary for balancing and healing
to take place.

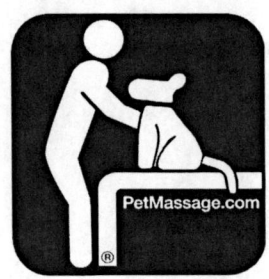

ART AND ESSENCE OF CANINE MASSAGE
PETMASSAGE™ FOR DOGS

ART AND ESSENCE OF CANINE MASSAGE
PETMASSAGE(TM) FOR DOGS

Contents

Introduction *4*

Influences and Development of PetMassage *9*
Two premises *10*
The author's story: PetMassage begins *12*
Epiphanies *18*
PetMassage evolves *23*
Influences on development of PetMassage *25*
Tribe *28*
Survey says *30*
About you *32*
History of massage *33*
Earliest animal massage *34*
The PetMassage School *35*
What you need *37*

Basic PetMassage Skills *39*
Skills *40*
Permission *42*
Touch, your touch *49*
You've got your whole world in your hands *52*
Pressure and duration *55*
Entering and exiting *59*
Palpation *60*
Breathing *63*
Palpable impressions *65*
Vectoring *68*
Tips for vectoring *76*
Touch with movement, the stroke *78*
Pushmi-pullyu *80*
Directions of strokes *82*
Connections *84*
Assessment strokes in series of threes *86*
Whose assessment *91*
Scratching *92*
Repetition *94*
Clasped hands *95*
Compression *97*
Joint mobilization *100*
Hey, hey. What do you say? *104*
Coming to terms with PetMassage *106*
Kneading *108*
Skin rolling *110*
I'll have that with a twist *112*
Muscle Squeezing *113*
Frictioning *114*
Tapotement -- percussive strokes *116*
Finger flicking *118*
Slapping *119*
Cupping *120*
Thymus thump *122*
Shaking *124* Rocking *125*
Holding patterns *128*
Reactive movement massage 131
Positional release *133*
Positional release:
Compression to expansion, demonstrated on an appendicular joint *134*

ART AND ESSENCE OF CANINE MASSAGE
PETMASSAGE™ FOR DOGS

Positional release:
Stretching to initiate recoil, demonstrated on the head, neck, trunk and pelvis *137*
Putting it together: the follow-on *140*
Feeling the love: shifts, internalizing releases *142*
Stretching *147*
Yawn *149*
Fascia *151*
Twelve body systems within the fascia *153*
Connect the dots 159
Grounding *160*
The post massage integration shake *162*
Body mechanics, part of body language *163*
Where oh where *165*
Safely assisting your dog onto and off the table *168*
Setting the scene: enhancements and distractions *170*

Putting it all together: Basic full body PetMassage *176*
A PetMassage session *177*
Elimination and hydration *201*
Thoughts and imaging *202*
Documentation *203*
Benefits for dogs *207*
Geriatric PetMassage Session *208*
Sports PetMassage *209*
PetMassage focus on the tail *212*
Focus on the neck *215*
PetMassage focus on the shoulder *217*
PetMassage focus on the hip *219*
When not to PetMassage *221*
Safety *225*
Humane Society story *227*
What are we not seeing? *229*

Your PetMassage *233*
Facilitating *234*
The role of presence *236*
You're the only one who can provide your PetMassage *238*
PetMassage Scope of practice *240*
The function of a mission statement *242*
The history in the dog *243*
What's next? PetMassage workshops, online courses and instructor training *244*
PetMassage for kids *250*
Lessons humans can learn from dogs *251*
Lola's story *252*

Additional information for your reading enjoyment *255*
Appendix 1 Survey: Job description for PetMassage provider *256*
Appendix 2 Fascia dynamics *263*
Appendix 3 Healing crisis *265*
References/Bibliography/Suggested Reading *267*
Glossary *272*
Index *289*
More fine PetMassage CDs, DVDs and books *301*
About the author *306*

ART AND ESSENCE OF CANINE MASSAGE
PETMASSAGE™ FOR DOGS

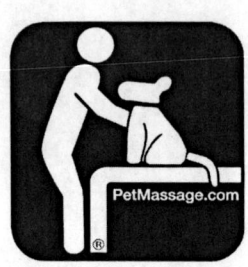

Introduction

PetMassage for Dogs, *Art and Essence of Canine Massage* may be the first book you read about canine massage. If you want to see if PetMassaging dogs would be a good fit for you, and this is your first toe in the water, I hope you find this series of lessons easy to follow, encouraging and inviting.

If this book is continuing education, you will see that PetMassage may differ from the human and animal massage that you already practice. *PetMassage for Dogs* is one of the texts for PetMassage Foundation level workshops and online courses.

PetMassage began by incorporating systems and techniques from diverse practices. It draws from Swedish massage, medical massage, sports massage, Healing Touch, intuitive shamanism, native/aboriginal culture, naturalist animal communication, animal behavior and old style, traditional veterinary practices. PetMassage continues to draw on the best of the old and the most effective of the new, forming a system that is compatible with, and that enhances, every size and shape of bodywork.

I recently had the opportunity to give a (human) massage to an elderly woman who had never had a massage before. She'd been experiencing cramps and numbness in her legs and didn't want to add any medications to the ones she was already taking ... especially pain killers and muscle relaxants. When her sister told her about the relief she's gotten with massage, desperate for relief, she called and scheduled her session.

When she arrived, my new client shared that she was confused and embarrassed. She wasn't sure what she was supposed to do. What happens during a massage session? How she was supposed to act? Was she supposed to take off all her clothes?

I knew that her inner verbal anxiety was so loud that she would be unable to hear any long explanations and descriptions. They would have made as much sense as adults in Peanut's cartoons, "Waa-waa-waa-waa." With confident body language and a few simple phrases, I was able to communicate through the din, that she was safe and in nurturing hands. She was confused. She could feel that I was showing my respect for her mind and spirit, as well as her body. I felt honored that she entrusted me in her experiment in this new avenue for her health and wellness care. I accepted the responsibility of providing her with the best experience I could offer.

This is just like working with dogs. They too don't know what PetMassage is, or what to expect. They might take one look at the table that we use for our sessions and tap into memories of angst-riddled experiences at groomers and vet offices. Again, I always acknowledge their anxieties and concerns. These are the filters through which they will perceive their experiences. I am always honored to introduce them to the world of PetMassage and the possibilities it offers.

My new human massage client, by the way, felt tremendous relief from her symptoms and anxiety. She was so comfortable with the process and my approach to helping her optimize her well-being that she continues to return for additional sessions.

My first massage opened doors between my body and mind that were longing to open. Under the slow, soft touch of my massage therapist, I drifted in and out of twilight consciousness. Concepts that I'd been questioning and meditating on fell together in ways that finally made sense. I left the table with a new understanding of myself and my place in my world. I discovered that I was able to work with people in more authentic and intimate (non-sexual) ways. In fact, the terms authentic and intimate took on more authentic and intimate implications.
I learned to connect, that such a connection was possible, spirit to spirit. And this was from one massage!

You can see that for me, my first massage was a life-altering event. I had been on a life-long quest to tap into my inner, soul-self. My goal was to discover who I was, what I'm doing here, why I'm living now, at this time, and find out if there were lessons I had to learn? Were there past life lessons and skills that I had forgotten? I had been on this quest from as far back as I could remember.

One of my childhood books that I studied, for example, was *Aesop's Fables*. I'd pour over the stories and their accompanying drawings. At seven and eight years of age, I was sure there were messages and hidden wisdoms there that I was not seeing. *Zen Flesh, Zen Bones* was another book I analyzed as a nightly ritual. Oh, if I could only hear my little hand clap by itself.

Now, with PetMassage, I have learned the lessons. I've accessed the forgotten skills. I have developed ways to open each of my clients, human and animal, to their healing potentials. I introduce them to their own intuitive, natural, and beautiful body-mind-spirit connections.

The stunning effects I experienced during my massage that afternoon clarified my personal philosophy and shaped my expectations for the experiences my massage clients could have; whether they are human, canine, feline or equine. Every PetMassage is an event that provides some sort of shift; a life-course correction.

It could be huge such as a geriatric dog who stops limping or spontaneously exhibits puppy-like exuberance. Or it could be so small as to be undetectable. To quote Sam Cooke's 1964 hit, "Yet I kno-o-o-ow a change is gonna come. Oh, yes it will."

This analogy applies: it only takes a plane taking off in Chicago a tiny variation in course or speed to make a big difference, on down the line. It could eventually land in Los Angeles or Seattle, or get there in four hours or six, or it might make several stops along the way.

I hold the same level of intention for you. Thank you for giving me the opportunity to help you shape your first impressions of canine massage, PetMassage for dogs. This book will be conversational; informal. I think that it is more enjoyable to learn new skills and new ways of approaching old skills, from someone who cares about whether or not you are "getting it."

I've been where you are. In my case, I can confidently use the term "clueless" to describe my approach in the 1980's when I started with bodywork on horses, and "clueless" again with dogs in the 1990's. You are surely further on in your life lessons than I was when I began.

In this book, we will discuss the basic skill set of hand positions, touches, strokes, and several manipulation techniques. You'll learn to incorporate your entire body; use all your senses--even some you may have forgotten you have -- to maintain your presence in the PetMassage "zone." You will learn the fundamental intentions of PetMassage, its history, uses, contraindications, and enough practical skills for you to deliver a confident, supportive PetMassage to your dogs.

PetMassage for Dogs will prepare you for the beginning massage sequence taught in PetMassage for Dogs Foundation workshop.

What kind of expectations can you have in studying this book? I cannot guarantee that you will enjoy massaging dogs, although I cannot imagine anyone not absolutely loving the experience.

I can promise that you will not be a PetMassage expert. Expertise in any new skill set takes time and experience. *PetMassage for Dogs* will give you a solid foundation, though. The techniques and theories offered here have been developed over a decade-long process of teaching over two hundred week-long workshops. You will find them very effective at helping dogs reestablish balance in their lives. And balance is what we are seeking. Balance creates happiness, health, and community comfort.

I can also promise that you will learn about yourself, your connection with dogs, and how you can help dogs discover their naturally intuitive, potential for wellness.

It would be pretentious to say that after you've completed this book, we'd be friends; or would it? Our conversation needn't be one-sided. I am available to personally address your questions and concerns through email. Write me. I'm looking forward to our dialogue. I'm at info@petmassage.com.

Influences and Development of PetMassage

Two premises

Dogs are more than our best friends. They are companions, protectors and comforters. Our dogs do more than greet us when we come home; they trust us and love us unconditionally. In return, we take responsibility for as many aspects of their lives as we can. We are concerned and responsible for them: body, mind and spirit.

To many of us, dogs are soul mates, trusted companions for many years. When I tell people what I do, I usually see a big smile and listen as they tell me, "I massage my dog all the time. She loves it; especially (pick one) when I rub her butt / squeeze her shoulders / scratch her belly / dig in around her ears."

Everyone has a naturally intuitive way of massaging their dogs. You already give basic massage to your dogs. It's a talent that comes naturally.

Does day-to-day petting count as massage? Massage in the broadest sense, yes. PetMassage? No.

PetMassage is a deliberate and focused skill set for touching your dog. It provides benefits to dogs that are so much more profound than they could get from affectionate petting, exercise or play.

In a PetMassage, each stroke is controlled in pressure, direction and intention. The pressure stimulates and affects the tissues of the body at varying depths. The direction stimulates or affects the flow of fluids within the body. And your controlled, intentional presence, stimulates and affects the way your dog's body responds. Your hands become finely tuned sensing devices, sensitive tools for assessment, support, realignment and reeducation.

You will learn to use your whole body In your dog's PetMassage – not just your hands. You become aware of your body's role as the connection between the energy, balance, and life-giving power of the earth and the energy, balance, and life-force of your dog. Your body becomes a conscious conduit through which the currents of healing, love, and life-energy flow.

Some of the many benefits of PetMassage are that it reduces stress, aids in healing and provides dogs the opportunity for ongoing internal self-reassessment and re-programming.

To give your dog the gift of PetMassage, is to reward him/her for a lifetime of companionship and friendship.

If you accept the premises that

    1) most diseases and dysfunctional behaviors are caused by stress, and that

    2) PetMassage induces relaxation and reduces stress,

you can join with me in understanding how PetMassage works.

The author's story: PetMassage begins

When I was five or six years old, our family took a driving vacation. For a week we meandered through eastern Michigan and southern Ontario and back to Toledo, OH. The second day of the trip, while we were having breakfast at a roadside diner, we learned about a mare who was just about to foal at a nearby farm. When we got to the farm, we were still in time to watch the little filly struggle and find her feet, and stand up on her rickety little legs. She was sticky-shiny, steaming and gleaming. Giddy feelings of witnessing a new life filled me. And on that crisp, sunny Canadian morning, I got hooked on horses. One of my all-favorite aromas is still horse manure.

My family always had dogs; one dog at a time. We could have more than one cat, but only one dog. When I was very small, our one dog, Dingo was her name, gave birth to eleven puppies. The space under our kitchen sink was the place Dingo chose as her birthing nest. One of them died soon after birthing. I imagined that it had come to our family as a mistake, so it turned around and went back to darkness. It was a non-issue.

So Dingo had ten amazing puppies to nurse and raise. When all those soft, fuzzy, warm, wiggly bodies crowded into that tiny nook to snuggle with her (that's what I thought we were doing), I was usually in there, too.

It was Springtime. When the back door opened for the puppies to be let out to play, out we'd all tumble, scattering onto the lawn. Bleary eyed with joy, we'd be mindlessly frolicking around on the worn patch of dirt where the grass never grew.

My favorite aroma is still puppy pee. And, lawns are still places to play. Perfectly manicured no-play zones of grass just don't make sense to me.

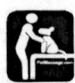

My other favorite aroma, while I'm on the subject, and jumping ahead in time twenty-five years, was my daughter's breath when she was a baby. Her tiny breath as she slept had the pure sweet fragrance of innocence. It's the bonus of breast feeding that dads can appreciate. It's a memory as sweet as puppy pee.

My experience with Dingo and the magnificent ten was short lived. I soon experienced the emotions connected with loss. Each day fewer dogs were there to play with. One by one, my little friends were disappearing. They were going to other people's homes to play with other kids. I was told that and I accepted that. And then, when there was only one puppy left, my parents announced that we were keeping the last puppy from the litter. We were a two-dog family. Yes!

The evening that the last of the puppies we were giving away had been picked up, there was a knock at our door. A mom was standing in the dim light of our entryway. She was sobbing. Her family's dog had just been hit by a car and killed. Her children were inconsolable. She was too. Her dog had been a black lab mix, just like Dingo. Was there any way we could part with either of our dogs? Please, *please*? My parents' hearts melted. And she drove off with ... Dingo. Joy, sadness; a "rolly"-coaster of feelings. And Peanut, the puppy was staying!

These were the days before puppy vaccines. Well, within a couple of weeks, Peanut got sick. Peanut died.

A short time later, we heard about a stray dog who'd wandered into a friend's yard. Watching the dog, he appeared friendly. Fifteen minutes later a tricolor beagle/hound mix with smiling big brown eyes came home with us. Pepper was my new awesome best friend.

Pepper! He was my advisor, teacher, confidant and all-around perfect buddy. We'd have unspoken conversations; what we now call animal communication. He was the one who taught me about body language. He taught me respect for personal space.

Pepper was a charming medium sized dog; maybe forty pounds. I later discovered he had every member of the family convinced that they were his favorite. He was the one who taught me to give compliments, always bring a present (even if it is a smile or a tail wag) when you are a guest, and to be considerate of other's feelings.

From the time that I first recall pulling myself up to stand, I had the intention to climb up onto a piano bench to play. Music is an important part in my life. I accepted intuitively that I already knew how to play. I felt I had had previous training from before I was this small child.

My music was pure passion and creative play. As a four or five year old, I would sit for hours at a time, creating interpretative piano soundscapes. I'd accompany whatever was happening outside my window: thunder, lightning, trucks and motor scooters, the rustling of trees and leaves in the wind, and rain (and more thunder). Then, of course, there were the birds and dogs, silently stalking cats, squirrels, chipmunks, and imaginary critters.

A favorite pastime was playing the same series of notes over and over ... and over, until I could detect the harmonics hiding within them. Dissonance to resolution. I'd sustain notes for as long as they were audible to find out what would happen to them. I'd follow on the shifting sounds, and draw new inspiration from the tendrils of echoes and their new beginnings of melodies.

That famous final 40-second long piano chord in the Beatles song, *A Day in the Life* revealed the same features. As we listened we felt the elements of the chord separate and trail off. They devolved into elemental traces of organic shadows of ancient memories. It was "a chord that seemed to fade away forever and leave you listening," in Jonathan Gould's words, "with a new kind of attention and awareness to the sound of nothing at all."

The residual harmonics would become present when the physical note evaporated. Exposed, they were allowed the opportunity to play with and form relationships with one another. Softly, timorously, tremulously. The intentions within the sounds eventually moved toward their potentials.

Sounds, vibrations, I knew, were more than what they appeared. I was not giving it much thought at the time. I was simply being myself and having a fabulous time playing with the piano. Sounds, vibrations, I knew, could unwind. They could optimize.

These concepts apply universally. When we are patient and wait; if we are quiet and observe, the over and undertones of the vibrations of everyone and everything around us will continue to resonate, eventually achieving closure and balance. It's the sound of one tiny hand clapping!

We all are more than what we present. We evolve and change. We all have the ability to unwind, to optimize and move toward our highest, greatest and healthiest potential.

As an adult, I reconnected with horses. Since the age of thirty, I've been a horseback riding enthusiast. Never happy flopping around in a big Western saddle, I was drawn to the style of horsemanship called centered riding, or dressage. My trail buddies who rode in big Western saddles used to tease me saying I looked like I was perched on a postage stamp.

It took several years to develop the skills of learning to coordinate my movements with those of my horse. Each ride was an exercise in reeducating my body. Initially, every positioning of my arms, hands, legs and heels were conscious decisions. Eventually, with repetition, my posture and movements toward balance became more automatic. I've always envied the riders who learned early and had been on horseback since childhood. Their intuitive movements appear to synchronize effortlessly with those of their horses.

My goals were to be able to ride balanced, gracefully and safely. Actually, to be honest, my biggest goal was to stay aboard the horse and not get my back muddy.

In centered riding, the one on top (me) needs to stay aware of how the one on the bottom (the horse) is compensating for the shifts he feels in the distribution of body weight above him. Lean forward and the horse moves forward to position his center directly below your center. Lean back and he slows down or backs up to readjust under your body. He positions himself where it is most comfortable for him, keeping you balanced and centered on his back. Shift to the right, he moves under you. Shift to the left … you get the idea.

As I became more comfortable in my seat, another way of saying, more experienced and intuitive, I found that my horse would respond, turning, slowing, stopping, backing up, and speeding up when I thought the directives. My thoughts appeared to be connected to the muscles in my legs and seat, shoulders, back and neck.

As they'd shift into the position for the movement, the horse would sense my redistributed weight. That was the only signal he needed to continue to stay comfortably under me.

We engage a similar interplay working with dogs, to achieve balance. Lean closer, pull away, turn to the right, or turn to the left. Work from above, work from below, work with the dog's head above your shoulder, or work with the dog's head below your armpit. Turn away; look away, cross your arms, cross your eyes. Every position you assume, each of your movements, shifts the relationship you are having with your dog. Your dog continually adjusts his position and posture to stay in synch with yours.

You work together in a kind of dance. Spooning each other's space. Adjusting your postures to each other, you comfort each other's physiological - social, emotional and energetic level.

In the process of becoming a Registered Nurse and Massage Therapist, I had extensive training in human anatomy, physiology, and patient care. The largest part of the caring process, I've learned, is listening, being completely present, empathizing with my clients and developing the ability to recognize their subtle cues. When I feel what my clients feel, I can be more compassionate, more understanding, more present for them. They feel more comfortable. They feel more accepted. When they are open to me I can be a better giver. They become better receivers.

One of the keys to encouraging openness, acceptance, and trust is being conscious of your body language. Our clients move to stay emotionally centered as we "ride" along together. Shift to the right, they move with you. Shift to the left ... it's the same concept.

These early experiences with the puppies, Pepper, the newborn filly, horseback riding, nursing and massage, were all part of my preparation for PetMassage. Either I just happened to have been exposed to a unique series of powerfully influential random events, or I could have been "meant" to have these experiences. Whichever I was experiencing, I was attracted to, good at, and excited about, a specific group of interests that when combined, determined the eventual direction of my life's work.

It felt then and still feels, as if there is a path on which I'm revisiting and expanding on known comfortable situations. Déjà vu awareness' used to be a rarity. Now, if I am not recognizing and remembering, it is unusual. The comfort zones I live and work in could quite possibly be the way to complete past--and continuing--life projects. It's a concept that gives a whole lot of meaning to life.

I've shared these experiences with you because in your own way, in your early history, you began preparing for PetMassage, too. Take a few minutes to recall all the people and situations that encouraged you on your path to appreciating, caring for and choosing to learn to massage dogs.

Just like you, I have spent most of my life seeking the answers to life's big questions: who am I, where do I fit in, is there a reason for my existence and if so, what is my purpose? My best teachers have been animals: dogs, cats and horses. They teach by example and express themselves clearer than we do with words.

The path I've taken began with the skills I brought into this life. There were some things I was naturally good at, things I readily understood. They were my talents. My basic skill set was augmented with life experience, traditional education, successes and lessons, and observation. Just like your path.

I discovered a powerful vision of how massage and bodywork can enhance the lives of dogs and the lives of the people who give it.

The lessons in this book enhance the bonds between human and canine. They provide a natural and fun way for you to give something very special back to your animals. The lessons are ones you can share, empowering other pet guardians all over the world to care for their dogs more effectively and responsibly.

ART AND ESSENCE OF CANINE MASSAGE
PETMASSAGE_{TM} FOR DOGS

Epiphanies

Two experiences profoundly shifted my life's direction. The first was a massage. The second was an Edgar Casey-esque awakening.

My first professional massage changed my life. I discovered that every facet of my life -- my body, my mind, and my spirit -- could be accessed and enhanced through this knowledgeable, compassionate touch. The tiny course correction that I made that single session dramatically altered the way the rest of my life would play out. It is the same with dogs. The tiny course corrections they make during their PetMassage effectively redirect and enhance the quality of their lives.

Since the early 1980's, I had been developing a personal style of equine massage techniques. In the spring of 1997 some of my more enthusiastic clients managed to finagle an invitation for me to give a demonstration of equine massage for an NBC television series called "Pampered Pets."

As the shoot progressed, the horse I was massaging closed his eyes and, immersed in his blissfulness, stood motionless. He was, one could say, baked. The horse was asleep. For all the action he was recording, the videographer could have used a still camera. There was nothing more I could do with him. With air time left to fill, my interviewer, a dog-person, turned to the camera and announced, "Dogs get stiff necks, too. Jonathan works on dogs, too." Out of the barn slowly trotted the barn owner's dusty "ol' yeller" dog.

I'd never even considered massaging a dog. I'd only worked with horses and bipeds, humans. I wasn't entirely sure what this would be like. I thought to myself, "This will be a challenge."

The camera rolled. I cradled the heavy golden retriever's head in my hands and watched his grayish-pink tongue loll out of one side of his mouth, dripping cool slobber on my wrist. Nice. The muscles under my fingers dissolved. His massive head sank into my hands. As his eyes rolled back into their sockets, to my

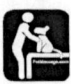

delight, I had a moment of surreal heightened awareness, an epiphany, that changed my life. It was on camera. I was at the right place at the right time with the right experience and my antennae just happened to be tuned into a very special frequency.

What I experienced was a vision that put everything I had ever experienced, and my quirky collection of traits and talents, in perfect perspective. What I saw opened my eyes. My soul remembered all the promises I'd made and the possibilities the future could hold. Visions are very exciting.

It was a spontaneous, profound; extraordinary insight.

For an instant, I was privileged to get a glimpse of a tiny aspect of the depth of it all. The veil parted and quickly closed back up again. This was the Akashic record that Edgar Casey had talked about. It is real and it is awesome. What I saw was more real than anything I had ever experienced. That instant, holding that old yellow dog's head in my hands, my heart smiled.

In a flash, I observed the full vision. I saw the beginning, the end, from the top and from the sides. Every image came at once, yet I could see, hear and know the story behind each detail. The narrow time-space I was working in, suddenly revealed its real self. It is deep, complex, clear and concise. It was a glimpse into alternative dimensions. They are always there. We must be just too busy in our flat earth life to see them.

The images validated all the knowledge and experience I'd acquired learning to help horses. And yes, now I could help dogs – specifically dogs -- and their people, men and women whose best friends are dogs. I could easily modify the massage style I had developed with horses, for dogs.

Mixed in with an enormous amount of information, I saw the covers of instructtional videos and books, the faces of hundreds of thousands of happy, enthuseastic people and even more dogs. People and dogs all around the world benefiting from courses I'm producing and teaching. Using the style of massage I'd soon call "PetMassage," pet owners, pet-care professionals, and my massage therapy colleagues would now be able to connect on deeper, more intuitive, and holistic levels than ever before, to help their dogs.

I saw the schools, the research, the international networking and more.

Following up on the enormity of what I witnessed in that split second, I was driven to spread the word about helping dogs and their people with massage.

Then, of course, self doubt crept in. Did what I had to offer add something or was I merely duplicating what was already there? What was the state of the art for canine massage? Did canine massage even exist?

ART AND ESSENCE OF CANINE MASSAGE
PETMASSAGE_{TM} FOR DOGS

There was research to do. I checked online. A primitive pre-Google internet search, under "canine massage" resulted in only a dozen hits. All of the other instructors who were teaching "canine massage," it seemed, had similar backgrounds to my own. The big difference was, they were working with dogs as a tangent to and derivative of equine and human Swedish massage. My focus was to be solely on dogs.

"The Equine Affaire," a huge horse exposition, was being held at the Ohio State Fairgrounds in Columbus OH the very next week. I needed to see who was doing what with dogs, so I attended.

I met most of the instructors there whom I'd read about online. To my relief, the massage form that I wanted to promote was not at all like what other instructors were teaching. The form I wanted to develop and teach had components and values that added to the field's knowledge base.

I was now comfortable, or at the very least, encouraged, to move forward.

Whoops. Now I had to develop a curriculum. Create the videos and write the books. This was all new territory for me. New and intimidating, this was all way outside my comfort zone.

Where to start? I contacted the folks from the TV station who had taped and edited the equine massage interview. We wrote a quick script, hired a videographer, located a professional voice talent, and met with two families with dogs. Within a couple of weeks we had shot over six hours of videotape of me massaging their dogs. We edited the tapes as if it were an hour TV show and my first professional quality canine massage video was "in the can."

I had 500 duplications made of the video. I purchased 500 video cases. I designed the video cover and had 500 copies of it printed in (woo-hoo) four-color. I assembled them in my living room. Videos, sleeves, and inserts were everywhere. My worktable was the top of my baby grand.

How to market them? We purchased a great domain name, www.petmassage.com. We created a simple website, and we put it out there. Then I sat back, thinking it was a job well done. The world would come rushing to my door...any time, now.

We shipped about a dozen videos in the first three months.

The extraordinary impact that I was expecting to make was disappointing. We had a few sales during the first few months. I started going to AKC dog shows as a vendor. The early shows were lonely. I was still a human-equine person, not a "dog person." My wife and I were still living in an apartment and had not yet adopted a dog of our own. My horse was boarded at a stable just outside the city.

People at the shows didn't quite know how to react when they met me. My energy was not yet at the frequency of "canine enthusiast." The concept of canine massage was so new that I heard "PetMassage? Does that mean you can teach my dog to massage me?" And, "I don't get massage for myself, why would I pay for my dog to get one?"

Every once in a while, though, trainers and handlers would surreptitiously sneak a dog to me if; especially when he/she wasn't moving quite right or was injured, or fearful or anxious. The dogs I massaged always appeared noticeably more balanced and comfortable.

As soon as each of the dogs dismounted (horse term) off my PetMassage table, they'd shake their little bodies vigorously, paws flying off the ground. I knew that to be a sign that they were integrating their freshly reengaged energy in their bodies all the way from their noses to their tails. I called it the "integration shake." After their PetMassage and integration shake, their movements were more balanced and their focus on handlers stronger.

Dogs that received PetMassage often won. Sometimes it was a class. Sometimes it was "best in breed." Every once in a while, "best in show." Handlers and trainers started seeking me out, reserving time for their dogs before they went into the ring. My favorite clients were agility and flyball dogs and their owners. A PetMassage for them could cut their times dramatically and enhance their safety. Some of the dog handlers were regular clients, too. They'd sit sideways on a folding chair while I used PetMassage techniques to resolve kinks in their backs and shoulders.

I was standing in my little 8' X 10' booth in Cobo Hall, at the Detroit Kennel Club show, when a young woman approached me, saying, "I have your video. I like it a lot." "That's great," I responded. "Who are you? I know everyone's name I've shipped videos to." She smiled and replied, "Oh, I got it from a friend, who got it from a friend, who got it … I think I'm around the sixth person to use it. We are all massaging our dogs the way you teach it. It is really helping them and I just wanted to thank you."

As she walked away, I visualized a map of the places we'd mailed our videos. We'd sent videos to most of the larger metropolitan areas of the US, plus more to England, Germany, Sweden, and Australia. I realized that we had been planting the first PetMassage seeds.

I needed a book to support the videos. (By that time we had created a follow up, second video, *Effective Pet Massage for Older Dogs*) I'd never written a book before. How does one write a book? Where do I begin? After many long nights, somehow, someway, following the outline and photos pulled from the videos, learning how to use the computer as I wrote, the book got written.

I had made a connection with another vendor at the shows who sold a huge selection of books. His books included everything you could ever want to know about dogs. We worked out an arrangement for him to purchase quantities of books wholesale and he generously invited me to be his guest, and be a draw with my book signings, at some of the major shows in the country including the Westminster Kennel Club Show at Madison Square Garden in New York and the huge Southwestern AKC Show at the AstroArena in Houston.

In 2000, Anastasia and I traveled to the UK, where I had the opportunity to give presentations to dog clubs in London and four arena scale demonstrations at the Crufts Show in Birmingham, England.

That first book is still a good basic text. It was written as an exercise for getting in touch with my heart. The difference between that book and this is a dozen years of experience, a dozen years of introspection, having written several other books, and videos, and of course, teaching over two hundred weeklong PetMassage workshops.

PetMassage evolves

Since the early 2000's, the art of PetMassage has evolved. PetMassage is not so much a technique as it is an art. A technique requires specialized rules and precise "mechanical" application. It is an art because it requires a greater breath of understanding and a flexible, creative, personally intuitive approach.

Dog's relationships to people are unique among all the animal species. The dog's role in the history of human civilization is astounding. We now know that without dogs, we homo sapien bipeds would never have progressed beyond groups of primitive hunter-gatherers.

In the past couple of decades we, as a culture, have shifted our view of the role of dogs in our lives. They had been considered as subordinate members of our families, albeit with most of the privileges, like sleeping in (the middle of) our beds and sharing our ice cream. The status and role of dogs in our lives are evolving and expanding. For people who have chosen not to have children, or whose children have grown up and moved on, they are filling a need for companionship. Dogs fill the void, emotional hole of loneliness. Eighty-five per cent of the dogs in the US sleep in their human's bed at night.

Dogs are often the social grease that helps initiate human relation-ships. It is no longer the school, the church, or the tavern where friendships are made. It's the dog park.

The more we learn about dogs, the more we appreciate their natural abilities, which can be enhanced even more, with additional training. Dogs are commonly used in law enforcement. They assist people who are blind and/or deaf; also people with epilepsy, heart conditions, COPD, Chronic Obstructive Pulmonary Disease, and who are unable to perform basic ADLs, Activities of Daily Living, by themselves.

Some especially talented dogs have been trained to sniff out early cancer malignancy and other disease forms as well.

Imitating these amazing creatures' remarkable abilities to hear and smell has allowed medical science and technology to produce new, imaginative, and innovative therapies. Even our medical tests are known as "lab" work.

Dogs are being used in correctional facilities' programs to help prisoners develop new skills and self esteem. Dogs are becoming important in elementary school reading programs. Children read to the dogs, who listen patiently and hardly ever correct the child's pronunciations.

Having studied "canids" for twelve years, I too have more of an idea of just how amazing our dogs are.

I now connect with dogs on a much subtler level. PetMassage takes me deeper than I could have ever imagined. My understanding of the potential of sensory perception and the role it plays, has increased dramatically.

The most developed evolution of the PetMassage practice includes the most recent advancements in understanding in the fields of animal to animal, animal to human, and human to animal relatedness.

PetMassage is the application of mind – body – spirit interrelatedness. It includes enhancing our own body awareness, and, from the viewpoint of quantum mechanics, understanding the power of witnessing. One student recently described our Foundation workshop as a "wisdom workshop."

Today canine massage practitioners are moving toward more universal acceptance. There is more consumer demand for PetMassage. It is now used as a complement to animal health care in veterinary hospitals. In kennels it is a specialized spa service. Our many graduates are now providing PetMassage to dogs throughout the US and in Tokyo and Osaka, Taiwan, Dubai, Manila, Mumbai, Sydney, London, Paris, Budapest, and Johannesburg.

We've seen this image, somewhere. It does sound familiar. Hmm.

Influences on development of PetMassage

The balance, movement, and body mechanics that are the backbones of PetMassage, were acquired through horseback riding and of all things, figure skating. Another powerful philosophical influence has been my long time practice of the martial art, Tai Chi Chuan. Riding for balance, skating for balance and movement, Tai Chi for balance, movement and body mechanics.

Another powerful influence came by listening to and learning from my wife, Anastasia. Anastasia has been a Rebirther, conscious-connected breathwork coach since the 1980's. Following the teachings of Leonard Orr and Jim Morningstar, the premise of her work is to use breathing patterns to reconnect with forgotten memories that underpin our current ways of interpreting our world.

Anastasia facilitates breathing sessions with her clients, supporting them as they work through their mind-body-spirit issues. Through this practice, they revisit memories of situations and people who might have been part of traumatic or transformative experiences, and experience the memory from the perspective of knowing, that they are in a time and place of safety. No one has to be the prisoner of their past. We no longer have to be victims. We can choose health. We can choose prosperity. We can choose happiness. We can choose to have choices.

Dogs, too, are often prisoners of their early training and negative experiences. We will learn that all of the perceptions of the memories of all of the dogs' experiences are retained in the connective tissue and nerve fibers. As the connective tissue is stretched and stimulated; as the synapses of the nerves are breached and strengthened, there are spontaneous releases of emotion and physical blocks. A large part of the art of PetMassage is acting as the silent witness for whatever the dog needs to emotionally process.

Anastasia is also an infant massage instructor, teaching parents to massage their babies. Following her, watching the interactions she had with babies, photographing her work for brochures, and listening to her teach parents, I began to view the dogs I was working with as develop-mentally stunted little humans.

Many of the observations of infant body language, I discovered, are the same as for canines. Human and animal body language uses the same signs and signals. Both are preverbal. Both are spontaneous and direct. Both are absolutely honest. Both are easily understandable.

Body language is our first language. We communicate to each other with shifting and posturing. As much as 80% of our communication with other humans in normal conversation is non-verbal. I learned that in nurses training. Body language has become a large part of the PetMassage practice.

Body language is our pets primary way of communicating with each other and with us. Words are unnecessary. Our dogs are constantly watching for cues that they can use to know that they safe, needed, and appreciated.

Most communication is unconscious. Some, as with centered riding, can be learned. If you are to be available and present with your dogs, you must learn to speak "body" consciously.

The next time you spend time with your dog, say, while you watch her inhaling her dinner, or when you're getting ready to take her for a walk, consider what message you are sending. What could she be reading into your posture.

See what her response is when you straighten your shoulders, or frown, or raise your arms over your head, or sit with your back to her. Notice how she reacts, such as cocking her head, shifting her weight, dropping her ears, moving her tail, opening her eyes wider, winking or lying down.

Ask yourself:
- What am I projecting by the way I'm standing or sitting?
- How is my weight distributed?
- Am I leaning forward, pressing into her space?
- Are my shoulders square to my dog, or are they angled off to one side?
- Am I pulling my upper torso back, away from my dog, or am I shifted to one side? Is my face angled up or am I looking down at the ground?
- Am I smiling or frowning?
- Are my fists clenched or are my hands relaxed?
- Are my knees locked or are they softly flexed?
- Are my arms or legs crossed?
- Am I breathing easily or am I holding my breath?

- Do my ears hang low? Do they wiggle to and fro? Can I tie them in a knot? Can I tie them in a bow?
- Your dog is watching and listening.
- What are you signing?
- What are you saying?
- What is she reading and hearing?

Tribe

It was at an esoteric massage therapy conference that I first experienced the concept of "tribe." My way had been a solitary one. Even in college, when the pressure was greatest, I'd never felt the need to join a fraternity. I was seldom in the presence of other people who shared my under-standing, or my passion for the big picture: discovering our place and purpose in the universe.

Working with fellow massage therapists, following the principles and practices of Orthobionomy™, I learned to be more observant, and sensitive to extremely subtle patterns of movement within my clients' joints, fascia and energy body. The spirit was similar to that of flowing with the tendrils of music when I was a child. It was similar to Anastasia's Rebirthing. Our empathetic bodywork helped our clients tune into their unconscious needs, fears, and intentions. It was all about tapping into the subtlest of cues.

Being with this group of people felt very familiar; kind of warm and snuggly. There was the faint aroma a puppy pee in the air. We recognized each other as if we had been together forever. Perhaps we had.

I had finally discovered my real family. This was my tribe! This tribe is not about heritage and blood lines. It is not about religion or ethnic culture. It is not about location, or generation, or any of the other attributes we think of when we think of "tribe."

If and when we are open and receptive, I remembered, reminded by my new family, we can participate in our client's healing process.

In the art of PetMassage, you will learn to internalize the sensations of patterns that you sense within the dog's body. This is the most effective way to track movements. Unravelings and releases. We'll come back to this.

At PetMassage workshops and IAAMB conferences (International Association of Animal Massage and Bodywork) I get to connect with and feel support from an amazingly talented, motivated and caring group of people. It is the strongest connection that I have ever experienced with any group. We share similar beliefs about animals. We have similar passions. Some are further along in their development than I am. Some are catching up. We are of one heart. We share the same soul. We are one tribe.

We know one another and are connected on a fundamental—a soul—level. My sense is that if you are reading this, you are a member of this tribe, too. Welcome. We've been waiting for you.

Survey says

PetMassage combines a broad range of skills and knowledge loci to augment your natural gifts. Several years ago I implemented a survey of former PetMassage students and colleagues in massage and bodywork. I was seeking to develop a "job description." The list of things we needed to know was extensive. As daunting as the list appeared, somehow, someway, we had all managed to develop the skills we needed to be able to practice professionally and effectively. [Appendix 1]

The survey also revealed something that was even more interesting. That is, we were all clearly and undeniably drawn to this field. We have a deep seated desire to help, comfort, succor, and heal animals. We have each developed our talents and skills to be highly individual and unique. We've also all taken unconventional routes to find our paths.

Many of us figured out later in life where our priorities lie, after moving on from other vocations. We may not have noticed it at the time; but, the work we were doing, was not fulfilling our emotional needs. Once we were introduced to PetMassage, we noticed. We stood up and experienced our own full body integration shakes.

We knew in our cores we'd rediscovered the path that was right for us. On the level of the soul, when we live, breathe, and work with animals, we are home. We are fulfilling our life's promise.

The skills were easy for us to understand and master. Learning them was less about entering into new, uncharted territory as about reconnecting with what we had known all along. Mastering skills we need is easy when it involves simply remembering. Everything comes naturally. The new expertise we have is in old skills we were already experienced in. When you already know where to focus, it is easy to learn and develop a practice. As we gain more experience in this time and space, we continue to grow and become even better at what we do and being who we are.

We were all predisposed to connecting with animals through massage and bodywork.

I have an aversion to the phrase, "it was meant to be." Perhaps though, we all were. Like petting the slippery newborn filly, snuggling with the puppies in the cozy nook under the sink, and tracking the shadows of sounds hiding in the piano, PetMassage is home.

About you

That's enough about me and my colleagues. Let's talk about you. You have always had a special connection with animals, too. Your course was clear. It is your past. It is your destiny. You were "meant to be" helping animals. You are the puzzle piece discovering its exact right place and position. Your joy, your obligation, is with animals. You've always known.

You have already developed your most important of the gifts just by being who you are. Interacting with dogs amplifies your frequency. You've done this, done that; worked this job and that job, studied and focused, succeeded or learned the lessons you needed to learn, and moved on. You've finally come to terms with the persistent question: what am I going to be when I grow up? The answer has always been there. Just in case you weren't paying attention. The answer is in the sound of your little hand. This is it: You will be who you are.

You've already realized that your love of animals is more intense than that of most people's. You are comfortable in dogs' presence and they are comfortable in yours. Petting and rubbing dogs, although fun, is no longer enough. You've realized that there is more you can do. You are pursuing important, valiant, valuable, and valued skills. You will help dogs discover their optimal potential with PetMassage.

PetMassage may be the vocation that is the most fulfilling for you. For you, the skills will be easy to learn.

Why is that? What creates this level of comfort? Why do you think you are drawn to PetMassaging dogs, while others scratch their heads asking, "Why would a dog need a massage?" and "Why don't you learn to massage people instead?" and "How do you even know if a dog likes it?"

History of massage

Some form of massage or "laying on of hands" has been used to heal and soothe the sick in every culture since people have figured out that touching makes us feel better.

To the ancient Greek and Roman physicians, massage was one of the principal means of healing and relieving pain. In the early fifth century BC, Hippocrates, the "father of medicine," wrote: "The physician must be experienced in many things, but assuredly in rubbing...for rubbing can bind a joint that is too lose, and loosen a joint that is too rigid."

Throughout the Middle Ages, due to the contempt for the pleasures of the flesh, there was little known of massage; until the sixteenth century, when it was revived, mainly through the work of the French doctor, Ambroise Pare. Moving ahead to the beginning of the nineteenth century, Per Henrik Ling developed what is now known as Swedish massage, developing his system from his knowledge of gymnastics and physiology from Chinese, Egyptian, Greek and Roman techniques. Swedish massage is still the foundation of the massage used in the US.

In Asia, massage has continued in an unbroken line since earliest times. Massage has always been more valued for its healing applications in the East than in the West. The poor country people in Asia were helped with "barefoot doctor" knowledge of Oriental medical theory, bone-setting and massage techniques.

Today, the therapeutic value of massage has again been recognized. It continues to flourish and develop throughout the world, both among lay practitioners and professionals.

Earliest animal massage

We know from Neolithic wall paintings in France that dogs and humans lived and hunted together as far back as 30,000 years ago. Dogs have been companions and hunting partners with man since the earliest of times. Bones of dogs have been found along with early human remains and other archeological artifacts. Dogs and humans have had a symbiotic relationship, each providing services to the other since the earliest of times. In return for scraps of food and shelter, (big sad eyes were begging at the table even then) early dogs would alert the early humans to danger and were invaluable helpers in tracking and hunting.

It is easy to visualize a cave dweller squatting on a rock in the circle of light around a campfire. She crouches, methodically rubbing her shoulder that has been bothering her. All mammals intuitively know that rubbing or putting pressure on a sore area eases the pain. She knows as well.

An injured dog limps into the circle of warmth and protection around the fire; comforted and attended by the compassionate touch of the caveman, medicine woman or cave kid. This was the first animal massage. It is the earliest, oldest, most natural and most instinctive self-health and animal-health care. It is still the most natural.

Massage for horses, dogs, cats, birds, reptiles, fish and all other living creatures has been practiced for thousands of years. Earliest written documentations go back 3000 years when Roman horse trainers and dealers described how, following established Greek traditions from a thousand years earlier; they would rub their horses to make their hides shine and to enhance their ability to run faster. These early writings were the formal guides of horse trainers and warriors for millennia.

The PetMassage school

In the US, several schools of massage for animals have evolved, each correct in its own way of approaching animals. Initially, the focus was solely on equine massage. Horse trainers, handlers and riders understood that their animal athletes would benefit from conditioning and "softer," non-medical, non-allopathic, interventions. They recognized that massage, was a drug free way to get their horses to move faster, jump higher, and have less down time due to injuries.

The primary form of massage taught and used by massage therapists for humans is Swedish. Human massage therapy state licensing is based on Swedish massage. Most of the animal massage instructors, having learned this tradition, are comfortable teaching variations on this form.

PetMassage, as a unique animal massage form, began in 1997, with the techniques of Swedish as a basis for its information and skills. This was the foundation platform from which we expanded using the techniques revealed in the epiphany.

As a PetMassage practitioner, you will use the same vocabulary to communicate as other animal care professionals. You must have a thorough grounding in western anatomy, physiology, and aforementioned Swedish massage theory and practice. It is valuable and relevant information. However, the practice of PetMassage is an art, and artistry comes in the creative applications of its skills.

The information in this text is the result of many years of practice and teaching over two hundred PetMassage for Dogs workshops. PetMassage is still evolving. Each dog I encounter offers new insight about dogs and about myself.

There is only one way to get to Carnegie Hall. It is to practice, practice, practice. PetMassage is a hands-on combination of skills that is impossible to learn, simply by reading a book, even this one.

I encourage you to move through this text slowly. Allow yourself the time to be reflective about whatever you read. Ask questions. Find out if this style of canine massage is a good fit with your personality. Pay attention to what is happening while your hands are on your dog.

Even at the beginning, novice levels, your PetMassage generates and facilitates powerful releases; releases intense enough to initiate dynamic course corrections in your dog's life. As you learn, and practice, you will develop muscle memory. The first time you attempt to do something it is always awkward and difficult. The second time it's a little easier. You know how it is supposed to feel. The third, you are even more comfortable. After a while, doing it is second nature.

As you think less about how and why and what you are doing, and having to execute each move independently, your focus becomes softer. Your practice will quickly expand to being more intuitively based. And the releases that your dogs experience will be even more profound. They follow your hands, reading whatever signals you emit. Dogs not only notice the pressure, the direction and the speed your hands are moving; they are aware too, of the confidence, the steadiness and the rhythmic flow from one movement to the next.

The history that you create for yourself and your clients, the proactive personal and political efforts you make, will help write the current chapter of the history of animal massage and the history of our culture. You are part of the continuum of a long tradition.

You've just shifted your course of learning, growth, and development. So, take your time. You will spend the rest of your life applying and tweaking your PetMassage with dogs.

The process is as important as the destination.

Unfasten your safety belts and enjoy the ride.

What you need

The keys to learning the art of PetMassaging dogs involve several aspects. One is to learn the manual skills. With focus, you will be able to learn these in a couple of days. These basic skills may be as much as you need or want to learn. They will be enough to get you to the point to administer an effective canine massage.

The elements that will add power and value to your work are the thought processes, the intentionality, the remembering, and your PetMassage body participation.

This is a short list of the things you need to get started.

- Willingness to learn
- Compassion
- Patience
- Open mind and heart
- Clean hands
- A body free of synthetic fragrances
- Ability to observe how your dog is experiencing your touch
- Willingness to learn to observe your own reactions and signals
- Quiet space, free of distractions from other people, animals, noise and aromas
- A defined space such as a grooming table or mat on the floor
- This book
- A dog
- Your dog's permission

Basic PetMassage Skills

Skills

The following is an outline of the most basic skills you will need to learn. We'll describe them, and discuss each of their variations and uses. You will learn to apply the essential breathing and body mechanics which will enhance your PetMassage. Then we shall put them all together in a canine PetMassage sequence.

1. Permission. You are entering your dog's world of personal space, body language, aromas, sound, sensation, and other unknown and unknowable stimuli and spatial references. Ask for permission to participate in their world and for them to participate in yours. Determine that you have received permission from the dog.

2. Touch is the purest method of connecting one body with another. Touch can be emotive, as in, "You've touch my heart with your words." Physical touch is your initial contact with the dog's body. Variables that affect touch are intention, mood, acceptance, your breathing, pressure, or depth, and touch duration.

3. Compression is the process of compacting the more superficial tissues against lower layers. Variables that affect compression include depth of pressure, duration, direction of force, placement of hands or fingers, student's head, neck and back posture, breathing and footwork.

4. Strokes, also known as *effleurage,* are touch with movement. Strokes, being the most like petting, are the most familiar movements we will be using. Assessment stroking includes noticing variations along the stroke path. Variables that affect strokes include depth of pressure, direction of movement, rate of movement, repetition, hand positions, the stroking technique, breathing and footwork.

5. Scratching and Frictioning stimulate the skin, hair follicles, and peripheral nerves. Variables that influence scratching and frictioning are hand position, depth of pressure, direction, rate of movement and repetition.

6. Clasp hands stimulates the nerves and muscles within and around the ribcage.

7. Petrissage, or kneading, the bunching up of the skin and coat, lifting it off the body and releasing it back onto the body, increases blood and lymphatic circulation within the deeper levels of tissues. Skin rolling stretches the skin, the fatty layer under the skin, and the connective tissue sheathes around the superficial muscles.

8. Joint mobilization stimulates and stretches the structures of the joint capsule, ligaments and tendons.

9. Percussion includes fingertip tapping, slapping, finger flicking, cupping and the thymus thump.

10. Shaking and rocking are more ways to mobilize and stimulate circulation and flexibility

11. Positional release involves all of the skills. It is the ultimate way to observe and support the dog's participation in PetMassage.

Permission

Before we touch any animal, or human, we get their consent. This sounds as if it would be obvious, yet we often forget. We see a dog and assume that they are having the same loving feelings as we have and go barreling right into their body space. Most of the time we are welcome. Sometimes, not. Just like humans, dogs have their aches, pains and weird moods. Just like us, there are times when dogs prefer to stay in their caves, and any touch, no matter how well intentioned, would be interpreted as an invasion or assault.

Dogs live in their personal space. A dog's perception of his space shifts and changes along with his moment to moment sense of safety, hunger, anxiety, health conditions, behavioral holding patterns, and moods. The size of the space varies with their moods and sense of empowerment. It could be one meter around them. It could be an entire yard. It could be held tight against their bodies. They honor their space, operate from it, and fight to protect it.

Ask for your dog's permission aloud. If you feel self-conscious asking in full voice, project your request as thoughts. Think it, as loudly and clearly as you can. Visualize a scene in which your dog is safe and enjoying your touch. She'll get the picture.

It is unlikely that your dog understands the words you are using. The largest number of words that any dog has been documented, through testing, to understand is around 300. It was a border collie [Morell]. Every dog, even those with limited vocabulary, will sense your intention. Ask the question. When you hear the words of what you are projecting you will know that the intention you are projecting is clear.

The answer may be yes; it may be no. Either way, you must be committed to honoring your dog's response. PetMassage is based on respecting your dog's needs. Your dog will communicate his openness to allowing you into his personal body-space. Your dog will not clearly state, "Why yes, that would be lovely," or "No, thank you, I'm having an ear wax situation and I 'vant' to be alone."

Read his body language for your answer. Body language is the combination of his intentional and unconscious movements and body positioning that projects a statement of purpose or intention.

His answer could be as simple as shifting his weight; giving *the suggestion* of leaning into your arms or shying away. The signs for acceptance or refusal are usually almost too subtle to notice. You have to learn what to watch for.

If your dog likes the idea, he'll make himself more accessible. He'll move closer to you; closing the distance between you and relaxing the boundaries of his personal space.

Shifting his center of gravity *toward* you indicates acceptance. Shifting his center *away* from you distances and is his signal for refusal. You knew these signs and signals already. You've been this way before.

If he doesn't want to be touched, he'll indicate through his body move-ments that his preference is for you to distance yourself. He knows it will take extra effort to reach him. And if you have to exert effort to do it, it will be less comfortable for you and less likely you will continue. If he doesn't want to be touched, his respiration will change. Compare your dog's rate and depth breathing when he is open and happy, to when he is closed and apprehensive. Openness has open breathing, closedness breathing is restrained. A "no" response will be contained. Breathing will be shallow and with hesitation.

You already know that when your dog assumes an erect stance (standing tall), holds the tail up or wags the tail in a slow sweep, and holds his ears pricked up, are all signs and signals. These may all represent confidence. They may not however, all be indicators of acceptance of massage.

The common signs and signals a dog uses to show fear or concern are universally understood and accepted by other dogs. Their body language communication is usually enough to keep them from having to confront other dogs. Postures that give the impression that they are smaller and less formidable, indicate that they are not a threat. No pack status can be gained by hurting a helpless little puppy in the dog world.

Submissive dogs present with a lowered stance, hold their tail down or tucked under, wag their tail quick and frantically; and look away, or turn their head to the side. This is animal-speak for not wanting to participate and not wanting to fight. [Rugaas]

The next time you are at the park, watch how a larger dog approaches a little dog when he wants to initiate play. He will lower his entire body, crawling forward on his belly, with his head at the same level, and his eyes will be looking up toward the little one. He may also quickly lick his own nose; a signal that horses and dogs use to indicate that they want to *join-up*, belong to a group or situation. [Roberts]

A shift of the light reflected in the eyes indicates you have the dog's attention. Watch for a quick glance and acknowledgement that you are sharing his space. This too, is a signal of acceptance. When a dog's pupils are dilated, however, it indicates that they are not willing to be clearly present.

Your dog uses his skin and hair to sense how safe he feels. Your dog also uses his skin and hair to broadcast his thoughts and emotions. Watch the hair on his back, neck and face. It is constantly shifting. It moves with his breath. It shifts with his moment-to-moment assessment of safety. The patterns and movements of the hair reflect his sense of control and how he is feeling. A softened coat along the topline indicates he senses no threat to his pack status and no threat with his acceptance of your touch.

When the hair lays relaxed over the skin, there is a slight lift in volume to maintain comfortable body temperature. A soft light bouncing off the coat indicates comfort in his body. It is a sign of acceptance. Slight changes in the sheen in the coat reflect slight shifts in your dog's comfort level. Large changes reflect large emotional shifts. A dog that is threatened will contract his coat tighter to his skin, as you might protect yourself pulling your sweater closer to your body when it's cool outside. Crawling inside the cave of his skin would make him appear smaller.

A stressed or anxious dog holds his breath, which swells his neck and shoulders. He will rise up on his toes. His forepaws will toe in, his elbows jut out laterally so that his pectoral muscles will open and not interfere with possible quick jumps to either side. Puffing up his chest makes him appear larger.

To another dog a puffed out animal appears to be a larger, more formidable opponent. This doesn't necessarily mean they will be aggressive; just that they need to be on high alert. Some dogs get "raised hackles" more easily than others; just as some people blush very easily.

Anxious dogs may experience spontaneous shedding, known as "blowing coat." Some dogs wick off dry, flaky skin similar to dandruff. His body appears larger because he is unconsciously tapping into his fight or flee response. This is the sympathetic nervous system's response to stressful events, preparing the body to defend itself or run to safety.

The fight or flee response is associated with the adrenal secretion of the hormone, epinephrine. It excites the body increasing heart rate, increasing blood flow to the brain and muscles, raising blood sugar levels, making the palms and soles sweaty, dilating the pupils, and stimulating the erector pili muscles of the hairs.

When a dog is stressed, the tiny arrector pili muscles at the base of the hair shafts shorten, they cause the hair to stand up, or move away from the body. The hair stands up in varying degrees all around the head and neck and over the topline, from neck to the tail. This hair pattern absorbs some of the light, softening the sheen. Light refracts off a coat stretched over muscles that are tense brighter than the light that reflects off a soft, relaxed coat.

An apprehensive dog will leave a trail of damp paw prints. If you notice moist prints on the surface where your dog is standing, see them as sweaty palms; a sign of generalized apprehension. Notice, as your PetMassage progresses, if and when they are no longer visible. This would be a sign of relaxation. Sweaty palms, we've just seen, is one of the fight or flee responses. Dogs release heat and fear by releasing fluids that can evaporate, through their saliva and in the spaces between the pads on their feet. The moisture in their paw prints is not just humidity. It includes oils with the scents of hormonal chemicals. Cortisol, for example, has unique chemical properties and reflects levels of stress and fear. Oxytocin, with its set of textures and aromas, reflects safety.

Dogs are not alone in this behavior. The signals we all use when we are ready to surrender or defend ourselves are universal. Horses flex the muscles on the sides of their necks, cats arch their backs, many fish can blow up to several times their normal size, and apes inhale and beat their chests. Trembling, sitting down, sweaty paw prints, holding the breath, racing heart rate, over-eagerness and rambunctiousness, all say, "maybe a PetMassage will be okay."

What if the dog you want to give a PetMassage is non-compliant? What if he is in pain, or obsessed with his own "issues?" What if he is scared or unavailable? What if you feel that working with him is a threat to you and your safety? What then? If you sense you are having difficulty connecting with a dog and notice resistance, you have to decide if you are the source or is it coming from the dog?

Nobody is equally comfortable with every breed of dog. I admit it. I have a preference for Boxers. There is just something about Boxers that makes me smile. Boxers and Dobies ... oh, and Weimaraners and Shepherds and Standard Poodles, Bulldogs, Pits, and Newfies, and some laid back small ones. I'm not a terrier person. I have issues about being told what to do and where to go, so border collies and Aussies who want to herd me, are too intense for my comfort. It is normal, and okay, to have preferences.

Our reactions to each dog are always biased. They are based on our memories of our emotional responses from experiences with similar dogs or similar situations. You may say, "I get along with all dogs and I don't have preferences." That is like saying you get along with all people, no matter what their personality or mood or familial relationships to you are. Most of the experiences we've had with most dogs have been wonderful. A few have been less than wonderful. A few have been scary.

We carry all of our memories and all of our responses in our unconscious. Our spontaneous responses are based in our histories. This is how we cope and how we survive. It is healthy.

An unpleasant encounter with the neighbors Chow Chow you had as a child, will continue its uneasy and apprehensive feeling throughout your life, whenever you are around dogs with similar characteristics, such as wooly coats or black tongues. Without realizing it, you wear your unconscious anxieties on your sleeve. You also project the loving times and generalized confidence with most of the dogs you encounter.

Every thought you have, whether you are aware of it or not, triggers physiological changes in your body. Each of your thoughts slightly alters your body chemistry, including the acidity in your perspiration. Just as dogs can read the characteristics of each others sweaty palm prints, they detect all our sweaty signals. They are all there; revealing who you are and why you are with them. Your fear/apprehension signals are in the aromas that make up your uniquely personal scent. You cannot hide it. It is impossible, especially from dogs. Your scents reveal your levels of confidence, fearfulness, anxiety, eagerness, hesitancy, tiredness, restedness, sickness, wellness, happiness, depression, hunger or satiety. They reflect your present quality of life.

Dogs can also discern what you had for breakfast two days ago and how well you are digesting it.

If your dog refuses to give permission, step back out of his space. Breathe. Realign your thoughts and clarify your intentions to yourself. Ask again when you are in a slightly different frame of mind. Your body language, breathing, dilated pupils, raised hackles, or head and shoulder carriage may have been the reasons he said "no." Your body may just not have asked right. Your body didn't say, "Please."

PetMassage requires a joining of like energies.

For some dogs, it may take more time to obtain permission than for others. With the dogs who are not quite ready and willing, take the time to establish trust. You must both be comfortable and feel safe with each other for the PetMassage to take place. If a dog is unwilling to receive a PetMassage gracefully, do not force yourself on him. There is never a time when a battle of wills is appropriate.

Permission is an agreement. Once you have asked for, and gotten, your dog's permission, you have a tacit contract: he/she will follow wherever your hands touch on the outside, from the inside. Your dog reserves the right to revise or negate the contract at any time there is feeling of disunity, disregard, or dissatisfaction.

Sometimes the answer is "no." The dog may be apprehensive, because he not yet know the joys of PetMassage. In his first session, then, you could spend thirty minutes in orientation, that is, developing trust and body-space comfort. If someone has brought their dog to you for massage, can you charge if he is not willing to receive? Absolutely. You are still using your skills of observation, assessment, animal behavior; all of which are part of the PetMassage skill set. Sometimes it takes multiple sessions just for the dog to overcome his fears and be comfortable standing on a table.

If there is ever a time when you feel fearful that you may be bitten, use the session for teaching the dog's guardian to massage him, demonstrating on a stuffed animal, and having her return demonstrate on your arm.

For the sake of moving on with the text, we'll accept that you have asked and you've gotten a "yes" response when inviting your dog to the dance. When a dog gives permission for you to participate in the PetMassage experience, he is declaring that he is accepting responsibility for everything that happens to his body, mind and spirit during and after his massage session. He is declaring his willingness to experience your responses to him, as well.

Your job is to then draw your dog's awareness to his body, and observe; encouraging him to restore balance and flow where indicated. You support him and any remodification that his intuitively reflexive body-nature chooses to initiate. It is the dog's PetMassage; his to accept, his to determine, his to experience, his to process and his to integrate into the core of his being. It's the PetMassage Hokey-Pokey; because, that's what it's all about.

Offering him the opportunity to give himself permission, you are bringing his attention to his body; his focused awareness to his generalized awareness. You are helping him to create an internal environment that is open and friendly to the potentials of balance and homeostatic healing.

PetMassage is most effective when it is wanted and the dog has an understanding that a special therapeutic event is taking place. Even if your dog gives you permission at the beginning of the PetMassage, he reserves his option to change his mind at any time. As you proceed from one sequence to the next, continue to reassess your dog's willingness to proceed, by getting his permission, throughout the session. Make sure that your dog is still with you in spirit and intent.

When you share your intention and presence you provide exactly what he needs. These are some variables that affect permission:

- the body space that you are creating with your thoughts
- your intention
- your mood
- your acceptance
- your breathing
- your confidence level
- your fears
- your dog's mood
- the dog's history with similar experiences
- the dog's personality, breed characteristics, age
- aromas such as perfumes, insect repellants, cooking odors, dusty carpets, mold, other dogs
- lights such as reflective flashes from passing cars
- sounds such as loud noises, high shrill children's sounds, deep rumbling thunder or trucks bouncing over potholes, other dogs
- the time of day such as dinner time or anticipated routine time of their person's arrival home
- the presence of their human guardian. Some dogs are more compliant, comfortable and better behaved when their pet parents are not in the room.
- the environment such as circulating fresh air, and open spaces

Touch, your touch

Touch is contact. Of all the senses, touch is the first to develop. As babies, it is the loving touch of parents that is essential to growth. In a study that I participated in with the Touch Research Institute, in Miami, FL, it was clearly demonstrated that premature, low birth-weight infants who received massage gained weight and developed faster than those in the group that did not get massage. Studies with infant primates have shown similar results. They show that physical contact is essential.

Touch deprivation, on the other hand, or rather, without the other hand, is physically and emotionally stunting. The absence of touch can result in failure to thrive in infants and in animals. There is a direct relationship between development and the quality and quantity of touch received.

Psychologists have proven that touch is a basic, essential need, just as food or water.

Touch is powerful. We all use touch instinctively, to comfort ourselves and those closest to us. Our natural response for bumps and bruises is to, "rub it better." When you have a stiff neck, you intuitively apply compression to it, and rub it. It is the same with a headache, a tooth ache, or a stubbed toe.

To touch is to connect. Touch can be physical, as in "I held your hand in mine." Touch can be emotional, as in, "Your words touched my heart."

Reaching out and touching others is a natural way to show our feelings; to demonstrate that they are loved, wanted or appreciated. Sympathy, understanding, and reassurance are all conveyed through holding, comforting, and stroking. Simply being present, sitting close to someone who is in pain is comforting. On the opposite end of the spectrum, when we're angry or frustrated, we also use touch; only in this context it is to lash out. Hitting, slapping, pushing, and restraining are also forms of touch. They are not part of PetMassage touch; but they are ways of touching.

PetMassage touch sends dogs the signals of connection, compassion, understanding, and support. The touch is therapeutic. It is awash with the intention to support their body's healing and rejuvenation.

Touching enhances your dog's self consciousness, his body awareness. He responds, observing his responses from within his body. Touch brings a sense of oneness; a sense of comfort and tranquility. The initial touching in PetMassage directs your dog's focus toward feeling how his body is interpreting the qualities and pressures he senses.

Your touch activates your dog's internal intelligence. It stimulates and circulates blood and lymph to encourage the release of endorphins, their naturally produced "feel good" chemicals, into their bloodstreams. Your touch even reinforces the work of cancer-fighting antioxidants in the blood.

Dog's bodies are intelligent. They naturally produce all of the chemicals their bodies need and have beautifully designed distribution networks. When there is an injury, the body can usually heal itself. If the body is stressed and needs to calm itself, or is sick and needs to combat germs or parasites, it can usually produce and deliver precisely the correct combinations of chemicals in the exact doses at the right times and by the precisely correct pathways to set it back in the direction of balance and wellness. It provides its own pain relief and regains impaired skeletal and muscular balance.

Most of the time your dog's body can take care of itself. Sometimes, though, it needs some help. *Your* controlled, skillful PetMassage touch is exactly the right way to remind their bodies of their power and potential for health.

Touch
- *enhances your dog's awareness of his body*
- *helps to distribute natural chemicals to calm and heal his/her body*
- *assists your dog in his/her natural abilities to relieve pain and discomfort.*

Touch, in PetMassage, is a physical and emotional connection *with no, or minimal, movement*. When you are still, your dog disconnects from his outward-focused, "chase reflex." His vision can be redirected inward when he is not looking outside. When are you most present and available for your dog? And when is he most present with himself? When you connect with his body and remain motionless. Touch in stillness, is called "still holding."

What is stillness? The qualities of your stillness are based on your unique life story. Your stillness is filled with the impressions of the shadows of your dreams and memories. These are the things that fill up the spaces between your thoughts. They form the matrix within which your thoughts move. Your stillness is filled with your body of knowledge. Your body holds your knowledge. It is the frame for your reference.

It is in the stillness within your movements where your dog's most profound connections and releases happen. Your response to the way your dog responds to you is based on the experiences that only you alone have had. And nobody can have had the exact same set of experiences as you. The stillness you provide is uniquely yours. Just as everybody has a unique fingerprint, everybody has a unique still-print. You have the particular quality of stillness that only you can create.

You are the only one who can create a relationship with you in it.

You've got your whole world in your hands

Your body chemistry, it turns out, in a complex series of feedback loops, controls the quality of your breath and the resilience in your hands. Each and every thought and feeling you have during your PetMassage affects your body chemistry.

With each thought and with the quality of each breath, your hands soften, tighten, dry, moisten, age or youth. The textures of your hands are dynamic. They are continuously shifting. The touch that your dog feels and responds to – your touch-print – (So, now you have a still-print *and* a touch-print.) is your authentic self, as you are in that moment.

When you touch your dog's body, not only do you feel it with your hands, you feel it with your heart. This is why it is imperative to stay very aware – very present – with what you are feeling.

As your persona experiences its moment to moment shifts, your dog is aware, responsive and adjusting to whoever and however you are. Does this mean you have to control your thoughts? No. It simply means that you are eminently readable.

What happens when you are resting your palm on your dog's shoulder, thinking about its texture, its warmth, how much you are into the PetMassage process ... and your cell phone rings. Your reflexive reaction is to withdraw your presence from your dog and move it to the cell phone. You must know who is calling. You haven't physically left; yet you have. Your hand is still on the shoulder. And, your dog has felt the disconnect.

Your awareness, your intentions, your responses to what you had been feeling were all radiating through the open lines and pores of your palms. When your awareness turned off, your hands closed up.

The blood that had been creating heat in your hands withdrew back toward your body, leaving them cooler, less responsive, tighter, and less interactive.

Correct hand position
Everything that follows depends on correct hand position. The position of your hands as you are touching your dog has a direct effect on how your touch is perceived. It, along with its pressure, movement, scent, and moisture, transmits the moment to moment level of your presence and connection.

Correct thumb position
Most of the time, your hands are held in a semi-relaxed position. Hold your hand in front of you, at heart level, with your thumb on top and your little finger below, just as you would when shaking hands or gripping a tennis racquet.

In this position your thumb is a natural continuation of the line of the bones in your forearm. A straight wrist is an optimal position in bodywork. It, along with a straight back, is a posture of strength and vitality.

Correct elbow position
Allow your elbow to hang easily; close to your side. This hand and arm position will keep your whole body engaged. It will also keep your arms down so that you do not reach your hands too far over your dog. Reaching over a dog's withers might be interpreted as a threatening gesture and could potentially shift the relationship your are developing into a different direction.

Correct palm position
Your palm is slightly stretched, as if you were holding a large sponge in your hand, and your fingers are relaxed and slightly curled. Maintain a straight, yet flexible wrist.

Correct wrist position
Whenever you bend your wrist to the point where you see the wrinkles of skin bracelets either on the front or the back, you are restricting the blood and nerve circulation to your palm and fingers. You are withholding important aspects of yourself when you cock your wrist: your presence and your awareness, and not allowing yourself to be fully available to support your dog's needs.

Within your body, all muscle groups are interconnected through a complex system of overlapping and interwoven grid of connective tissue, fascia. The movements that you make, or restrict, with one part of your body affect the rest of the body.

For example, turning your thumb down, flexes your forearm muscles, rotates your triceps, presses your bicep muscles into your pectorals and pulls the skin on the side of your neck down toward your chest. The skin on your neck pulls the muscles on that side of your face down.

Continuing, turning your thumb down pulls the sides of your mouth down into a frown. The skin around your eyes sags, giving you a droopy countenance. Frowning and droopy eyes both cause a rise in blood pressure and trigger your body's feedback loop. Your system receives a jolt of compensating release of steroids to bring your body back to harmony. Your dog can smell the steroids of your frown. Frowning, droopy eyes and the smell of fresh steroids are signals dogs read as danger.

Even in ancient Rome, the signal for life and freedom was thumbs up. The signal for death and "bad luck" was thumbs down. Think about all that your body is signaling.

Most of us have two hands, so if one hand has reached as far as it can and is turning over or bending, so that your thumb is beginning to point down, switch hands, and complete the stroke, by turning your body and completing the stroke with your other hand, picking up where your first hand ran out of arm.

In your PetMassage you will be using every part of both hands. You'll use the fronts, sides and backs, fingertips, thumbs, and knuckles. Throughout it all, you will continue to signal "life, liberty and the pursuit of happiness" with your thumbs. Right? They will always be on top.

As long as you keep your wrist flexible and straight you'll be an "understanding listener and straight shooter."

Pressure and duration

We will use only these three main descriptions for the depth of PetMassage touch. Of course there are nuances, such as light-medium, and medium-firm, and firm medium. There is firm-firm, firm to medium light; and we could go on. We'll stay with these three:

        Light (presence)
        Medium (firm contact)
        Deep (pressure)

        Light is on the skin.
        Medium is in the skin.
        Deep is beneath the skin.

Light touch
The depth of the light touch is minimal. Your hands are simply present. They barely graze the uppermost layer of your dog's coat or skin. Light touch pressure would be about the weight of a dry washcloth -- a thin one.

Even at this lightest of caresses, *especially* at this lightest of pressures, there is a lot going on behind the scenes. You and your dog both continue to experience the many textures and patterns that your share. You both become aware of each others temperature, openness, and resilience.

On the conscious level, you notice the characteristics of your dog's hair and skin. He senses the same set of qualities in your skin. On the unconscious level, your body is having an ongoing dialogue with his body. On this level his body notices all the shifts of oily information-laden moisture in the whorl patterns on your fingertips.

Light touch connects with the skin and coat. It stimulates a flood of awareness', both of the current situation and of the memories of the dog's recent experiences. When it snows, the coat gets cold and wet.

As your still-hold continues, you and your dog move into the intimacy of your shared moment. You both become more and more present; more aware of yourselves, more aware of each other.

Think of moving into a darkened room after being in a bright hallway. As your eyes adjust to the dark, shapes that you'd been unable to distinguish begin to emerge. As you stand there, more and more distinct features become visible. In the dark, we see with an entirely different set of rod and cone receptors in our eyes. We also use a complementary set of sensory skills; one we forget we have except when we use them.

With your hands on the dog, with patience and stillness, you begin to notice the unnoticed levels of movement. There will be tiny shifts and contractions; twitches and releases. The fascia beneath the skin is constantly moving. It is readjusting and realigning. You will also sense subtle variations in textures, densities and temperature.

This level of touch may not feel very effective, when you are begin-ning your practice. We as a culture are used to exerting a lot of pressure to make things happen. We need to feel that we are in control. We are physically causing something to happen.

Your dog feels every one of these light touch sensations, too. He takes them as cues for the direction of his own bodywork.

Exercise:
Sit quietly, with one hand resting lightly on your forearm. Notice the contour of your arm as your hand molds around it. Observe all the sensations that you feel. Notice the temperature, the texture of the hair, the resilience and tonicity of the skin. Close your eyes and experience the connection your hand is having with the arm.

Shift your attention from your hand palpating and experience your arm experiencing your hand. Notice the shapes of the fingers, the spaces between them, their textures, resilience, tightness or soft-ness. Notice the palm. Does it feel soft, firm, dry or moist, heavy or light? Are you feeling more weight or pressure from a particular area or is the pressure consistent? Can you sense the creases, or lines in your palm? Heart line, Fate line, Life line, Head line, Chorus line?

Notice if, as the receiver, you feel any emotions that stem from this prolonged touch. Does it feel comforting, restricting, smothering?

Return your awareness to your palm. Do you sense any difference in how it is assessing your arm, now that it is aware of what the arm is experiencing?

Medium pressure
Touch at the medium depth provokes reflexive contractions of the muscles just beneath your dog's skin, his superficial muscles. The pressure of "medium pressure." is about the weight of a wet wash cloth. At this level, you will notice another set of textures, such as skin tags, bumps and nodules on, and beneath, the skin. You can also discern the quality of your dog's pulse and the general contours of larger muscle groups, joints, and bones.

You will notice the qualities of the superficial layers of fat and you can assess the qualities of vascular and lymphatic circulation.

Deep pressure
Press with a little more pressure. You are at "deep pressure" now. Deep pressure is still not very heavy. Pressing in with "deep pressure." has about the weight of a wet hand towel.

You have entered the level for a set of deeper textures; the shapes and tightness of larger muscle groups and attachment sites, tendons and ligaments, the shapes and resilience of the ends of bones at joints, organs, breathing patterns, and deeper body rhythms.

This level accesses your dog's strongly held beliefs or physical holding patterns. These include congenital diseases and tendencies, cultural breed memories, and chronic conditions. These memories, these behavior patterns, held within your dogs DNA can be accessed with deep touch. They all have the potential to be reeducated, transformed and corrected.

On each level, and especially the deep level, PetMassage can affect the most strongly held "core" beliefs and conditions.

Review:
Light
With the lightness of a feather your hand softly brushes against the surface of your dog's coat. Pause and observe. Even with this lightest of pressures, your dog will be able to feel your hand. Dogs feel mosquitoes when they land on them. If they have that degree of sensitivity they *will* feel your hand. Take several long breaths,
continuing to pay attention to what you are feeling. When you sense that you have as much information as you can get at this point, or you get bored or anxious, increase pressure to medium. FYI: dogs can smell boredom, too.

Medium

The amount of pressure for medium would be the same as you would use when rubbing your eyes. Medium pressure is plenty. It is simply the weight of your hand resting on your dog's body. It is still pretty light pressure, compared to the pressure that you might expect in a human massage therapy session. Remember that dogs are not humans and that they live in a world of subtlety and nuance. Take several long breaths, continuing to pay attention to what you are feeling in your hands. When you sense you have as much informa-tion as you can get at this point, increase your pressure to deep.

Deep

The amount of pressure for deep would be the same as you would use when you rub your fingers firmly over your forehead moving your skin back and forth. It is still not very much pressure. On your dog, the pressure would be enough so that you can feel the characteristics of the ribs and muscles beneath the coat. Once you are accustomed to the new depth with its unique set of textures and sensations, breathe and observe. Compare this to scuba diving. Every 30 feet deeper you go, the temperature is noticeably cooler. The amount of illumination you have to see is different. And the habitats are home to a particular set of critter species.

Deep pressure for dogs is less intense than deep pressure for humans. People have a lot more tolerance for pain and can justify "exquisite pain" if there is the promise of relief afterwards. Dogs live in the present. They are not going to wait around to see if it is a good hurt, a bad hurt or it will ease up after awhile. "Exquisite pain" is a concept dogs cannot wrap their minds around. To a dog, if there's pain, it's happening now. Now is all there is. And, the only thing that is important is that the pain goes away.

When we are learning PetMassage we all have a tendency to want to use too much force. We project that dogs would appreciate the same kinds of pressure that we like to feel. Yes, your dog loves a vigorous rubdown. Yes, he gets all excited when you dig deep into the muscles around his butt. And yes, this very deep work can be part of his full PetMassage experience. However, your use of excessive force might inadvertently hurt your dog.

Your dog will not tell you. He is enjoying your undivided, one-on-one attention. He may think you are playing or he's getting some rough and tumble affection. Your dog will probably be fine. He is all forgiving for any errors in judgment you make while you're learning. That's what unconditional love and understanding is all about. In time and with experience you will develop subtlety and restraint and learn to appreciate "exquisite gentleness."

Entering and exiting

Once you and your dog have made a connection, you will feel your hand being pulled in and held, as if by a Star trek tractor beam. Your dog's bio-magnetic energy field is synergizing with yours. He will hold your hand in place until his body has completed the work it needs to do. Then, you will be released.

Both you and your dog work together, synergistically, to create movement. Your dog determines the rate of movement, when to release your pressure and the direction of your retreating hand. Allow your hand to be guided out from his body.

The transitions from light to medium, medium to deep, deep to medium, and medium to light all flow one into another. Occasionally, there will be an abrupt change in character. Once you initiate a still-hold, do not intentionally change the amount of pressure to deeper or lighter. Think your hands to be at the level they need to be and, observe how the dog's body pushes and pulls them where they need to go.

Your hands exit your dog's body-space by riding his thought currents, his willingness or resistance, coming off his body. When withdrawing your hands from your dog's body, pull them out slowly, in stages, pausing and acknowledging at the medium level, and then pausing at, and acknowledging, the light level. This will be more comfortable for your dog, who is closely following every move from an inside, aisle seat. Visualize the hands of a pianist completing his recital. They float up, rising off the keys, trailing after the fading final notes.

Exercise in observation
Compare and contrast the textures you felt as you were moving in, as you revisit their habitats at each level on the way out.

> You and the dog are both assessing.

Palpation

A palpation is defined as "an examination using fingers." It is "a method of clinical examination using gentle pressure of the fingers to detect growths, changes in the size of underlying organs, and unusual tissue reactions to pressure."

We have a new interpretation of palpation as a result of incorporating hypotheses from quantum mechanics that suggest that whatever we focus on, expands. The simple process of touching, combined with observing what you experience, or, witnessing your touch, just by itself, is already having an affect.

As you increase your awareness of the sensations you detect in your fingers and hands, your dog becomes even more aware of his own body's presence.

Every touch your dog feels expands his experience of his body.

Dogs are hard-wired to be attracted to and follow movement. They are emotionally stimulated by movement. This is the "chase reflex" and its name describes exactly what it does. The quality of movement, or lack of it, either calms or stimulates. Fast stimulates. Move your hands quickly and you increase excitement. The slower your movement, the less your dog is stimulated. Slow hands calm. Still hands give dogs the opportunity to go within; to focus inward instead of on whatever activity is going on around them. Since most dogs are motivated by movement and pressure, long duration, light, still holds may induce your dog to forget that you are there. That's highly unlikely, though.

Your dog's most powerful experiences with textures and sensations will be when he can stop reflexively chasing your movements; when you pause. You both can observe and experience within your stillness's.

When I was just sixteen years old, I had the good fortune to meet a Master. He was the famous big band drummer, Gene Krupa at Krupa's Jazz Club in

Manhattan. He was a legend. I was awestruck. My brother played the drums so we had his records at home and had listened to his playing. When I told him how much I enjoyed his work he asked me to come up to stand next to him and his drums. He leaned forward and shared a secret with me. "Listen to the spaces between the beats," he whispered. "That's where the music is." Your magic is also in your "paws" between your strokes.

Take your time. Move slowly. Give yourself time to adjust your inner vision. Think about what you are feeling. Immerse yourself in the momentary experience. Feel what you are thinking. Process spontaneously. Quick patting cannot possibly have as profound an effect or result as purposeful touching.

Palms
The most responsive parts of your hands are your palms. Your fate, heart, love, and prosperity are all revealed there. I know this is true because when I was around four years old, a gypsy in a little shack at a roadside rest stop outskirts of Carlsbad, California, told me so. In his mysterious wisdom, he also foretold that I would be an adult when I was grown up. Everyone makes mistakes.

The honesty and truth that we find in nature are reflected in the unique character of the lines in our palms. The uniqueness of our hands is meaningful and offers lessons that resonate with authenticity. For millennia, hands-on healers have relied on the information they sense through their palms. Healers have developed the ability to project the energy of their intention and redirect the forces that they feel. They palpate the universal life force, the Ch'i, the energetic stuff that creates life, through their palms.

Exercise
Stretch your hands as wide as you can. As you widen your palms, the shapes, the calluses, the muscles, the skin and the feathered lines in them stretch. Observe how the lines expand and contract when you move your little finger up and out; and rotate your thumb.

Although it seems counterintuitive, you get more fundamental information through the palms, than with the fingertips, which detect fine detail. Your palms are the direct link of your dog's inner movements to your body's core.

Just as importantly, your hands reflect your moods, your attention, and your breathing. Your palms telegraph every tightness and tension, softness and comfort, you are holding in your body.

Your palms must be ready to be sensitive to whatever they touch. Your palms are the outermost extremities of the large bones in your body.

- Keep your palms slightly taut, yet relaxed.
- Keep your wrists, finger joints, and hand muscles soft and relaxed.
- Keep your wrists, finger joints, and arm muscles soft and relaxed.
- Keep your wrists, finger joints, and shoulder muscles soft and relaxed.
- Keep your back and spine straight, yet soft, relaxed, and flexible.
- Keep the back of your head lifted so that your chin is slightly lowered.
- Keep your pelvis tilted up, so that your back is straight and you are concaving around your abdominal core.
- Keep your knees slightly bent soft, and relaxed.
- Breathe through your nose. Keep your mouth closed. Maintain a gentle contact between the tip of your tongue and the roof of your mouth just behind your teeth.
- Maintain an even cycle of breathing, making sure that you do not get short of breath. If you do get out of breath, you are no longer fully available for your dog. Pause, focus on your breathing until it becomes quiet and even. Then continue.

Observe and feel
- your dog's response to your touch
- your reactions to your dog's responses
- your thoughts and feelings that surface

Anything that restricts your breathing reduces your ability to feel.

Breathing

Have you ever been in a stressful situation and someone coaches you to *hold* your breath? Me neither. Incorporate and integrate conscious breathing into your hand movements, your arm movements and even your footwork. Your touch and stroking will be magnified.

Quiet breathwork is essential for a successful and de-stressing PetMassage. Whenever you begin a session, pause and take a minute or so to observe and regulate your breathing and heart rate. If, at any time during the session, you notice that you are out of breath or that you are moving too fast, simply pause. Consciously observe your breathing.

What if your breathing is not in a balanced and rhythmic pattern?

Consider what happens when you forget to breathe. Holding your breath cuts off essential oxygen to the cells that are keeping your hands alive. The cells immediately begin to atrophy and your body initiates mechanisms to protect itself. One of the ways is to pull the blood from the periphery to the vital organs in the core of the body. When the tissues in your hands tighten, you are sending signals to your dog that you are stressed, traumatized, scared, angry, or distancing yourself for some reason.

In the canine world, dogs react just like humans when they are stressed. They prepare to either fight or flee. They tense their muscles. Tension in your hands, may be interpreted as stress or anger. On the other hand, when dogs sense soft and relaxed hands, they respond in kind, by relaxing.

Incorporate your entire body with your breath. Visualize yourself standing in a swimming pool, with your knees slightly bent. The water is at your shoulder level. As you inhale, feel your body buoyed up so that your legs straighten and you are rising up onto the balls of your feet. Allow your eyes to gently close. As you exhale, allow your eyes to gently open and as you feel your body deflate, soften your knees, and feel your weight fall back into your heels. Inhale up. Exhale back.

Repeat, breathing through your nose, incorporating a Buddha smile. It's the smile in which only the edges of your lips turn up.

This Tai Chi exercise moves the breath in 8 directions. Observe how you feel during and after you've repeated the sequence several times. Stand, with your feet shoulder width apart, your knees soft and slightly bent, your spine straight and your hands hanging softly next to your hips.

1. Gathering (inhale) Scoop up the energy around the fronts, sides and behind your hips with your hands. Bring your hands to center, below your belly button, palms facing each other, holding the energy between them.
2. Moving up (exhale) Extend your hands to the front. Raise your hands to heart level, palms facing each other, holding the ball of energy between them.
3. Expansion (inhale), Spread your arms out to the sides, your ball has expanded and is now huge. Embrace the energy.
4. Contraction (exhale), Bring your hands together, compressing the energy between them. Extend your arms in front of your heart.
5. Pulling in, withdrawal (inhale). Direct your palms toward your heart and pull the energy into your body.
6. Pressing out (exhale) Rotate your palms to the front, and press your hands forward to a stretch at heart level.
7. Lowering (inhale) Slowly allow your arms and hands to float down. Your palms hover over your Lower Dan Tien, below your belly button. They bring the energy of your body with them.
8. Releasing (exhale) Allow your hands to relax and open comfortably at your sides. Observe the energy as it flows out your fingers into the space that surrounds and supports your body. The energy, channeled to the ground, stabilizes and grounds you.

Notice that when you inhale, you rise up onto the balls of your feet and when you exhale fall back into your heels.

It is impossible to synchronize your breathing patterns with dogs. Their respiration rates are very different from ours. So, breathe comfortably at your rate. Observe your dog breathing comfortably at his. It is not the rate that is important. It's the comfort.

> Your PetMassage palpation is a way to get a sense of how the entire body is functioning.

Palpable impressions

So now you are comfortable with asking permission, touching, and breathing. Your breathing presses your body and hands into your dog's body-space. Your breathwork raises your hands, lowers your hands, pushes your hands, and pulls your hands back to you.

Pay attention to what you sense as you slowly enter and retract your hand from your dog's body. What do you sense when you are still-holding your dog? What do you sense when you are pushing and pulling your hand across your dog's body. And while you are moving your hand, and keeping your dogs attention, what are you supposed to be observing?

What are you looking for? What are you assessing?

During assessment, you observe not only the unusual "news" that jumps into your awareness because of its strangeness. You observe the beautifully functioning, healthy aspects of the body, as well.

You will usually feel harmony, balance and healthy muscle tone. Sometimes other textures, body tissue behaviors, present themselves. They may declare themselves as tightness or knots in the muscles, warm or cool areas, and changes in texture patterns of the coat. You may discover lumps, bumps and pockets of soft, squishy fat under the skin. You will also take note of any tender spots or unusual patterns in the hair.

Let's look at what you may discover:

Muscle tightness is common. Muscle tightness stems from incorrect skeletal alignment or any discomfort, which would lead to your dog restricting his/her own movements to guard against pain. Muscle groups all have attachment sites. These are their beginnings, origins, located proximally, and where they hook onto, the insertions, located distally. These will tell you what the actions of the muscles are and how they relate to other muscle groups that are also involved in their movement.

Actual "knots" are rare in dogs. Knots are caused by the bunching up of fascia, the connective tissue in and around muscles, in the attachment site. Overwork, injuries, strain or muscle spasms could all be reasons the fascia might have gotten stuck and lost its elasticity.

Warm areas could be signs of bruises or areas of infection where your dog's blood has pooled beneath the surface of the skin. Warm areas are found at injury sites as part of the natural healing process. Whenever you sense heat you are aware of the miracle of natural healing as it happens. At joints, when there is a sprain (tear) or strain (stretch), the joint capsule (that encases the ends of the bones, ligaments, muscles, and other cushioning elements) produces additional synovial fluid that increases the pressure within the joint. The extra pressure, part of the process of inflammation, is what creates the heat in swollen joints. The fluids in the joints bathe the tissues, and restrict movement. Any large movement will apply pressure to the nerve endings and cause discomfort. It is the body's own system to naturally discourage movement when time is needed for healing. Our dogs' bodies have the marvelous ability to heal themselves.

Cool areas are often the sites of old injuries, or surgeries, where there may be incomplete or reduced blood circulation to the site, or stagnation of energy flow. Around the cool areas, the blood and lymphatic fluids have devised collateral, alternative, routes to access and nourish the distal (further from the heart) tissues.

Lumps and warts are common in older dogs. They often are superficial and benign. If you notice any changes in lumps and warts from one PetMassage to the next, refer your client's caregiver to their veterinarian for advice. You may be detecting a symptom of serious disease. This early detection often becomes apparent with long-duration still-holding and is one of the best reasons to PetMassage dogs.

Fatty pockets under the skin may be just fat, but then again, they could be indicators of other health problems. Bring these to the dog's caregiver's attention. Encourage them to keep a vigilant eye on these areas to watch for any changes. Many of the changes we're referring to are not really measurable; except that you will note "a change." That's all you need to do. Assess them, note them, keep an eye on them, and if they change, tell the caregiver to ask her vet.

Tender spots will be readily apparent. Your dog will let you know when you touch an area that causes discomfort. He will mouth your hand when you are near areas that are causing him concern. He will move away from you, yelp, snap, or collapse away from the pressure. You may be stimulating acute bruises, sprains or injured tissues. They may also be sites of chronic discomfort such as arthritis or hip dysplasia. Mouthing, or holding his mouth on your hand while you are touching him is also a normal puppy behavior.

Uneven hair patterns, whorls or cowlicks (caused by hair follicles that grow at odd angles compared to the rest of the hair of the head) indicate an imbalance in blood flow to the area beneath it. Not enough nourish-ment is getting to the skin and hair. This, too, should be brought to the caregiver's attention.

> Uneven hair patterns or cowlicks may indicate underlying tissue is out of balance. The tissues are not getting the nourishment they need for optimal health and function.

Vectoring

Vectoring is an important element in the PetMassage form. It is a means of observing how the dog's body responds to various pressures and touch patterns. Vectoring is a systematic sequence of still-holding two areas of the dog's body at the same time and observing the musculo-skeletal movements under your hands in the channel, or *vector,* between them.

When executed correctly, PetMassage Vectoring can provide everything that is necessary for a great body, mind, and spiritual experience. It is comforting to the dog, giving him an opportunity to experience his body in an emotionally and physically safe environment.

His responses to this still-holding touch are significant. Observe using the inside of your palms. Notice any movements that happen in the body between your hands.

Still-holding draws the dog's attention to five specific fascia meridians, or vectors on his body. You both have the time, space and opportunity to observe body patterns and rhythms.

As you hold each vector, visualize the waves of the ocean lapping up onto the beach washing the rocks with foam. Each wave retreats back into the water, leaving a shimmering lacey residue. In its wake, you see all the small rocks and shells repositioned in the sand. Then, caught by an inflow of the next oncoming wave, part of the water as well as the debris suspended in it, is carried back up onto the beach. The new waves push through the resistance and create new patterns.

Your hands have an effect similar to the waves, except they are clean and dry and they can do more.

Your hands can feel. They can detect tension and discomfort. They can orchestrate change. They have the power and capacity to influence the circulation, muscle tone, balance and quality of harmonics of whatever is within them. They can assist the dog to create life style course corrections. Your hands are an extension of the earth, itself.

After we've gotten our dog's permission, use the following specific order of six still-holding PetMassage vector patterns at the beginning and end of each PetMassage.

Hold both of the areas at the same time in the exact order as described.

1. Chest and middle of the back
2. Withers and croup
3. Both hips
4. Both sides on the ribs just behind the elbows
5. Belly and back
6. Repeat the first one: chest and middle of the back

Place your hands on your dog as demonstrated in the following photos.

Take your time.

With each still-hold, take at least three, long, deep, unhurried breaths from your belly. Hold each vector for as long as thirty seconds, or until you sense that your hands are being released. Then it is time to move on.

> PetMassage vector patterns are most effective in the order that follows this specific pattern of fascia meridians.

1. Chest and middle of the back
   Place one hand on the chest, cupping the breastbone in your palm and your other, dorsal hand, the one on top, on the spine over the ribcage behind the withers.

   Between your hands are the contents of the ribcage. You are containing the heart and pericardium, the lungs, and the lymph nodes on the underside of the spine in your hands.

   Hold your hands in place for three long breaths: inhale, exhale… inhale, exhale… inhale, and exhale. Observe the textures of hair, the temperature of the coat, the consistency of the hair, the resiliency of the tissues beneath the coat. Note any movements that occur between your hands. Feel the heart beat. Feel the gentle expansion and contraction of the chest with the breath.

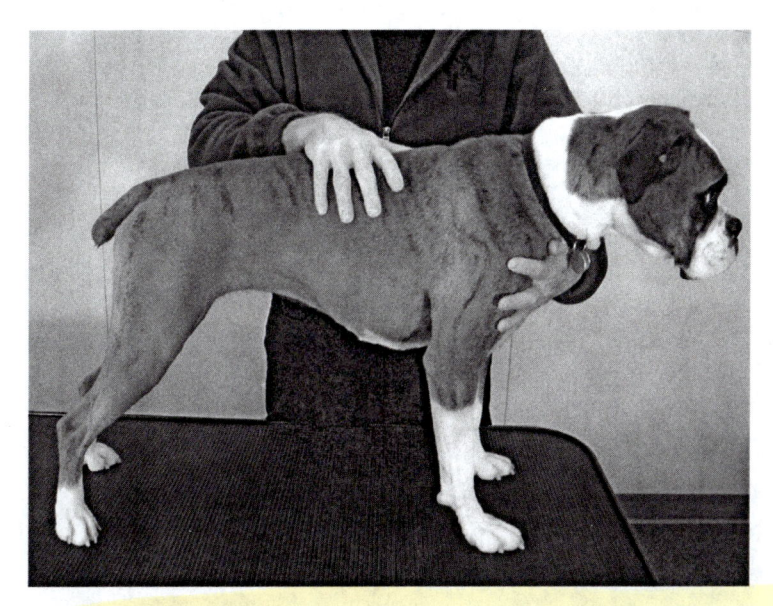

   Good. Now, without losing contact, slide your hands into the next position.

> Lifting both hands off is your dog's signal that the session is over and he/she can leave.

2. Withers and croup

Place one hand over the withers, the area on top of the shoulder blades just behind the neck and the other on the croup, the section on top of the pelvic girdle that angles back toward the tail. Between your hands runs the thoracic and lumbar spine, all the ligaments that hold it together and provide its support, the muscles that provide its movement, the pathway of the Central Nervous System, and a long series of lymph nodes on the underside of the spine. Any and every stimulation, any and every movement you notice is affecting all of the above.

Keep your hands quiet and still. Watch the tissue move between them.

Maintain contact with your dog with at least one hand, throughout the PetMassage. Lifting both hands off disconnects you from your dog. It signals him that the session is over and he has permission to leave.

Maintain your still-hold on these two points for at least three long breaths. Then, slide your hands down to the next position on the hips.

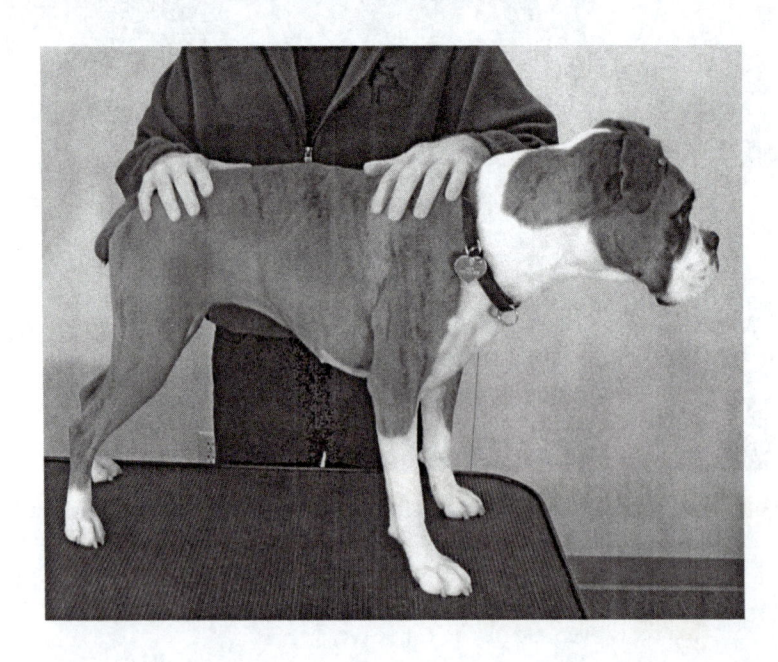

3. Hips

Place one palm on either side of the hips. To locate the hips, follow the contour of the femur, the long upper bone of the hind leg, up to where it articulates with the pelvis. You will feel a little bony knob through the muscle. Cup both hip joints in your palms. In your hands are the vulnerable hips, the hip ligaments that provide support and the origins of the hip muscles that provide movement.

Envision the contents of the hips between your hands. You are holding the three bones of each side of the pelvic girdle, the ilium, ischium and pubis. Passing through the pelvic girdle is the caudal (tail end) of the spine: the lumbar vertebrae, sacrum and the coccyx bones. Ligaments attach these bones to one another and tendons hold muscles that provide movement to the bones. Within the pelvic girdle are the organs for reproduction and elimination.

This is all pulsing within and against your palms.

Still-hold, breathe, and observe.

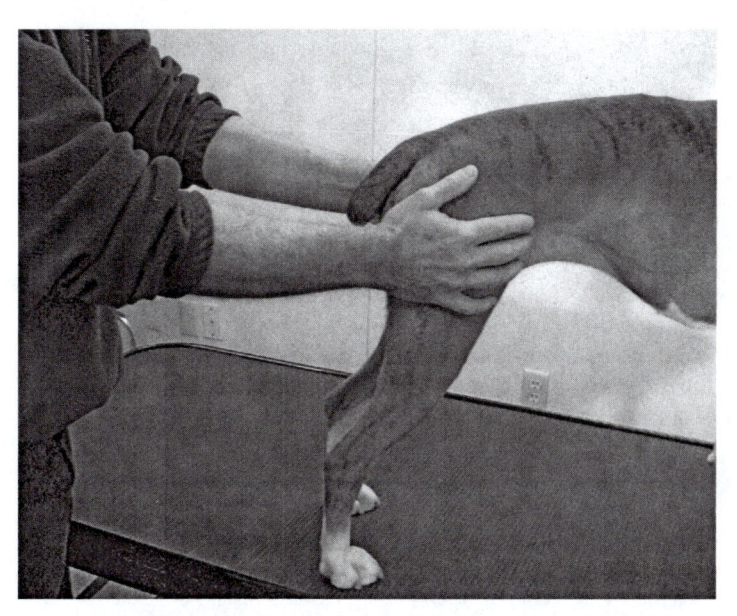

After completing the hips, slide both your hands cranially, toward the head, up the sides, onto the ribcage for the next vector position.

> Close your eyes.
> Observe your breath for three long,
> slow cycles.

4. Heart to heart: hands on ribs
Place your hands on either side of the ribs just behind the elbows. You are cradling the contents of the ribcage: heart, pericardium, lungs, and esophagus. In this position you will be able to feel the heartbeat and the ribs move in and out with each of your dog's breaths.

Breathe, relax and observe.

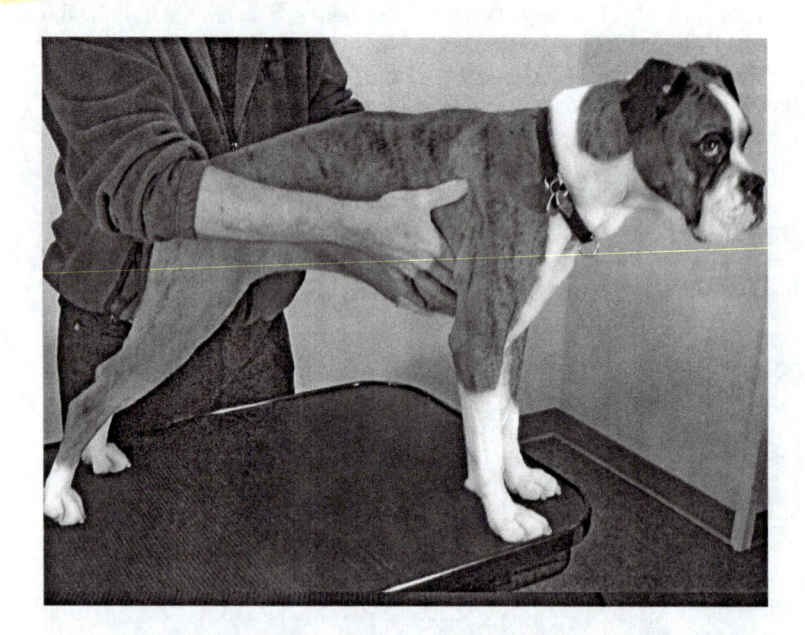

Slide your hands around so that one hand is cradling the belly and the other is resting on top of the spine right in the middle where the thoracic vertebrae transition to the lumbar.

> Whenever you are not sure if you are using too much pressure, use the Rule of Halves: decrease it by half.

5. Belly and back

Your hands are positioned so that your dorsal, upper hand is on the middle of the back and the ventral hand is cupping the belly. Your dorsal hand can feel the little dip in the spine on the mid back, where the thorax transitions to the lumbar. Your dorsal hand is containing the middle of the spine with all its ligaments, muscles and lymph nodes, the CNS, Central Nervous System that flows through the spinal cord, the caudal area of the lungs, the kidneys, adrenal glands and intestines.

Your ventral hand covers the caudal part of the ventral ribcage, and the xyphoid process, the little bone at the bottom of the sternum. Within the costal arch is the soft underbelly containing the diaphragm, the liver, the spleen, the pancreas, the stomach and the small intestines. Your hand is supporting the body's processes of digestion, absorption, and elimination. The stomach is intimately connected to the dog's emotional responses to stress, the Limbic System. Still-holding gently stimulates and supports the nerve plexuses in this area. Breathe three times, relax and observe.

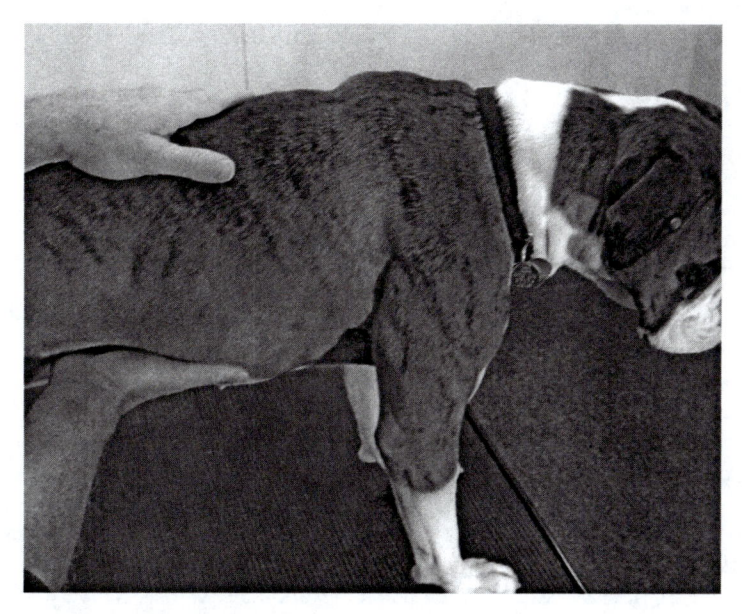

Are you noticing that you dog has different shades within the colors on his body?

Are you noticing variations in texture?

Complete the Vector series by bringing your dog's attention back to where you started. Keep the dorsal hand in the same (mid-back) position while sliding your ventral hand onto the sternum, the breastbone.

6. Chest and middle of the back

Breathe, relax and observe the movement within the spaces between your hands. In your mind's eye, without moving your hands, review what you have just experienced. Has your perception of the dog's body changed? Is the dog more comfortable with you now, than he was at the beginning of the vectoring sequence?

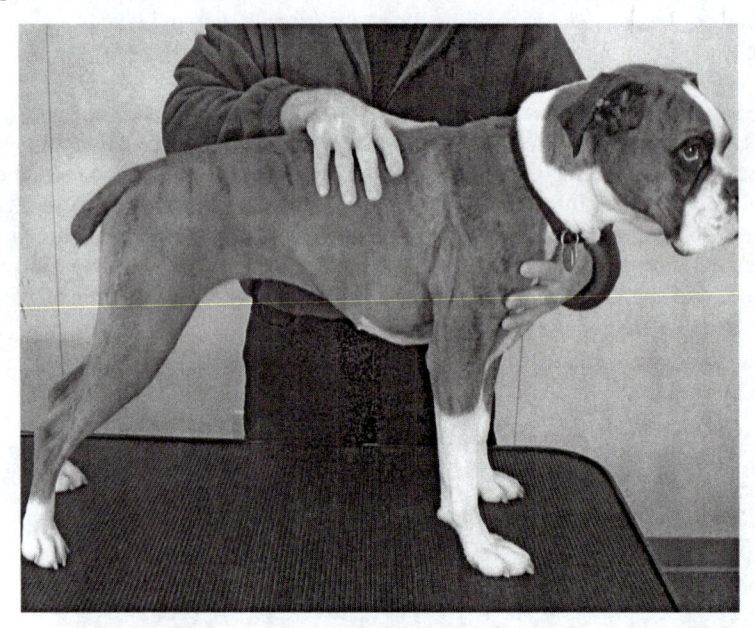

Practice this series, several times until you have trained your body to follow this specific order. The more you practice, and the longer you stay within each vector, the more you will be able to support your dog's experience. Vectoring is active observation. It is intervention through observing, asking permission, assessing, opening, aligning, *balancing, supporting the inner healing, closing and thanking.*

Pay close attention to any movements you sense in the coat, skin and superficial muscles under the skin. When you palpate, the tissues shift, slide, and revolve; when you feel tightness dissolve, when tension evaporates, you are actively participating in the dog finding his balance and harmony.

Tips for vectoring

Hand positioning
Your hands and wrists need to stay in a comfortable position so that good blood circulation to them is maintained. When you are comfort-able the fascia that is responsible for the coordinated movement of the tissues in your hands, wrists and arms, is open.

Soften the muscles in your palms. Allow your whole hand to mold itself into the contours and shapes of your dog's body.

Body mechanics: positioning
Drop your elbows so that they rest easily against your sides. There should be no tension in your upper arms and the pectoral muscles on the sides of your chest and beneath your armpits.

Soften the muscles in your neck and shoulders. If you feel tightness creeping into your neck muscles, lift your shoulders up to your ears, hold, and allow them to drop back down. Breathe and observe. Watch and enjoy. The show is a sensory deluge.

Vectoring, by itself, can give you and your dog physical and emotional feedback, for support, and re-education. The body moves against your hands and back into itself as did the waves.

You can return to the comfort and understanding residing in the gentle focus of vectoring any time during the PetMassage.

Whenever you are not sure what to do next, or if your dog is becoming anxious or uncooperative, breathe, vector with stillness and observe.

Practice the points on this list to enhance your experience during vectoring:

- Keep your hands and fingers still (no movement).
- Keep your hands and fingers quiet (no talking with your hands).
- Keep your thumbs up and your little fingers down, like you're holding a tennis racquet.
- Focus your attention on your palms as they rest comfortably on the body.
- Notice how the pads of your fingers sink into the hair.
- Notice your breathing patterns.
- With each inhalation, feel your body buoy slightly up onto the balls of your feet.
- With each exhalation, feel your body drop back into your heels.

This is a review of variables that affect touch, palpation and vectoring
- intention
- mood
- acceptance
- your breathing
- pressure, or depth
- touch duration, the length of time you linger on each area of the body

Touch with movement: the stroke

Thank you for your patience, so far. You have probably been more interested in learning the more active movements of PetMassage: the pushing and pulling, twisting and percussion. When we think about massage, these are the movements we visualize. They are all import-ant, too. And, they are all rooted in the deep, quiet communication that is in still-holding.

These are the fundamentals. Everything in the rest of this book is predicated on your understanding and ability to practice permission and touch.

Now you can start moving touch across the dog's body.

Strokes are simply touch with movement.

The stroke is the most like petting. This is what we intuitively do when we want to comfort and soothe our dogs. While stroking can be part of petting, petting is not at all the same as stroking.

You will hear this often: "I pet my dog all the time. Is this the same as massage?" Again, the big differences between petting and the PetMassage strokes are that you are:

1) being purposefully aware of what your senses detect, and
2) fully responsive to all the subtle ways your dog is responding to your touch, and
3) skilled in the use of several techniques, knowledgeable of their affects and responsible for their correct and appropriate applications.

The long flowing stroke, known as effleurage, has a different purpose. While petting expresses affection, PetMassage effleurage expresses support of your dog's potential for wellness. Stroking incorporates your personal investment, intention, presence, awareness, as you and your dog focus on the qualities of the textures you palpate.

Touching with movement gives you the ability to notice variations along each stroke path and within each level. For example, you may not notice that an area feels warm unless it is a variation in a cool path. Or, tissue may feel soft, and puffy only when it is compared to other areas that are more toned.

Your hands and fingers are in the same semi-relaxed position that you used with touch.

Body mechanics
Allow your wrist, elbow and shoulder to stay relaxed, too. The whole hand to shoulder apparatus should work as a unit and can have only minimal movement within it.

As you pull your hands over the surface of your dog's body allow them to softly collapse, conforming to the contours on the body. Again, your pressure and primary connection is through your palms. Your fingers either guide the way, clearing a path for your hands to follow or trail behind, depending on whether you are pushing your hands away from you or pulling them back toward your heart.

Turning your body will be the impetus of pushing and pulling your arm and hand over the dog.

Effleurage:

a light, gliding motion over the skin that always maintains contact and directs the stroke away from the heart, moving with the lay of the hair. This stroke is frequently used at the beginning and end of a massage treatment to invoke soothing and relaxing.

Pushmi-pullyu

Strokes go in either of two directions away from you, and toward you.

Core values
Your arms and hands and fingers are extensions from your core. Your core, where your abdomen and diaphragm are, is where your power lies. This is where you hold your intention, your compassion, and your intuition. You breathe from your core. You feel your emotions in your core. You react from your core. Your PetMassage relationships spontaneously process through your core.

The movements of your hands and arms always begin in your legs and torso.

Integrating your legs into each of your movements is the first step in being able move from your core. To turn your core, you must transfer your weight from one leg and pivot onto the other. Shifting your center of balance naturally rotates your waist. It is impossible to move from your center without engaging your pelvis. As your waist and torso turn, your arms follow. The Tai Chi exercise of transferring your weight and turning is helped by visualizing rotating a potted palm back and forth, leaves following the movements of the stem.

The flow of movement in your body moves like a string of pearls. This is another well known Tai Chi analogy.

Exercise Earthbound
Visualize yourself standing with your feet shoulder width apart, your knees soft and slightly bent, and your spine straight. Step back, catching the full weight of your body with your rear foot. Your heel, pressing down, secures and stabilizes your connection to the earth.

Beneath you, planet Earth throbs with power and life. Earth's awesome power moves up to support your foot and body. Each time you drop back into your rear foot, you get recharged, re-grounded and re-stabilized.

Feel your rear foot collect the Earth Chi. Transferring your weight to your forward leg and step forward. The Chi follows the shift of your center of gravity and flows up, filling your pelvis and abdomen. As you continue to turn, it continues to move; up your spine, through your shoulders, arms, and hands. The power of the earth is the energy that is propelled out your palms and fingers.. Everything is attached and coordinated, just like a string of Chinese pearls.

Power is not generated from movements of your shoulders, and they do not stem from the muscles in your chest. They are all the result of your footwork. Shifting your weight onto the front foot, stepping forward, projects. Projects what? It projects your intention, your power, your Chi.

Each stroke originates from the center (core) of the Earth and its power reaches up through your body to connect with your dog.

Coordinate your footwork with your breathing. Inhale when your hands move into your body. Exhale when your hands move away.

Exercise
Extend your arms and hands heart high in front of your shoulders, palms facing each other. Your thumbs are up. Your palms are slightly stretched and your fingers are relaxed. Think of your arms as branches on a tree. To move your hands, you must move the branches. To move the branches you must turn the trunk. To turn the trunk you must transfer the center of gravity from one set of roots to the other.

Plant your feet so that they are stable. Turn your torso, shifting your weight from one leg to the other. When your shoulder pulls back, as an extension of your spine, your arm and hand come along with it. Look straight ahead in the direction you are now facing. Keep your arm outstretched in front of you.

To pull your hand toward you, turn. Twisting your torso pulls your shoulder, elbow, wrist and hand across your body. To push it away from you, turn. Your whole body movement pushes and pulls your shoulders, arms and hands.

Directions of strokes

The direction of the stroke determines its function. The directions of strokes are described in three ways:

- flowing with the lay of the coat
- against the lay of the coat
- across the lay of the coat.

Your hand glides easily and smoothly over the surface of the coat when it moves in the direction of the lay of the coat. Your hand moves from the front, cranial (head/cranium), of the dog to the tail, caudal (tail/caudad), and from the dorsal (top side) down the legs to the toes, ventral. Your dog's arterial blood flow, from his heart out to his extremities is the same. When your hands move with the grain, you are smoothing the coat. You are reinforcing normal cardiovascular circulation. This has a calming effect.

Strokes that flow against the lay of the coat will cause the dog to look ruffled. Instead of relaxing the skin and the dog within, it stimulates. The coat will look confused and excited, and it has the same affect on the dog. These strokes move in the direction of the venous blood flow, from the extremities back to the heart. Strokes against the lie of the coat have the effect of encouraging your dog's blood to circulate back to his heart. And this supports the body's natural inclination toward homeostasis.

Stroking perpendicular to the lay of the coat is also exciting to the tissues. Stroking across the coat warms the tissues and enhances muscle tone. These movements push and pull the fascia beneath the coat, stretching it, increasing blood circulation.

Notice the specific effects each stroke direction has on your dog's body.

- Strokes moving away from heart, with the lay of the hair, are relaxing.
- Strokes moving toward heart, against the lay of the hair are stimulating
- Strokes across the lay of the coat are exciting. They are called cross-fiber strokes. They can break up muscle knots and dissolve trigger points.

Combine the strokes that move up, down and across with your body movements. Shift your center of balance, turning your arms with your torso with each compression and release.

Strokes can be with the hair, against the hair, or across the hair. Strokes can be light, medium and deep pressure. Stroke on all three levels:

> Light is on the skin.
> Medium is in the skin.
> Deep is beneath the skin.

Breathing mechanics
As you exhale, your hands become heavier and drop further into the body space of the dog. Pressing in, focuses your dog's attention on that area and stimulates it.

Inhaling, lightens your hands and ever so slightly, pulls them from your dog's body. Your dog continues to follow every gesture and every intention. As your hands pull away you draw your dog's body awareness with you. It is relaxing. This is a powerful way to discharge discomfort, tightness, any imbalance you sense.

A variation of the stroking hand position is to curl your hands into loose fists. Pull your knuckles across the body, leaving a wake of furrows behind your hands. Push through the hair, leading with your knuckles, opening a path for the backs of your fingers and nails. This position offers a different quality of sensation. It will be much more stimulating than working with the palms.

Connections

Each and every one of the billions of inner body connections (the cells, nerves, muscles, tendons, and organ systems) has the potential for moving toward its own place of greater comfort…to discover or create more balance and a better quality of life.

Your PetMassage has an affect on all these connections.

Each connection has an awareness of
- comfort or discomfort
- flexibility or inflexibility
- stability or instability
- and connection or disconnection to its intuitive nature

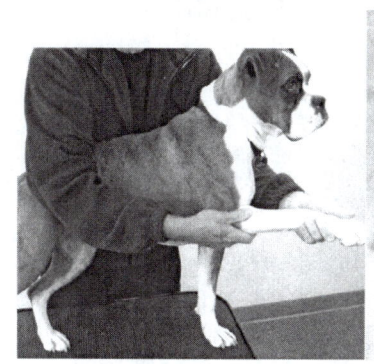

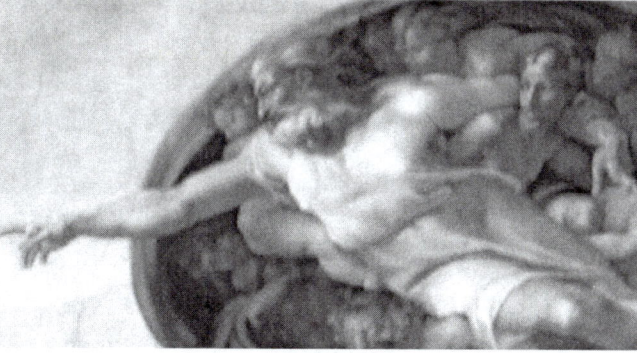

Processing

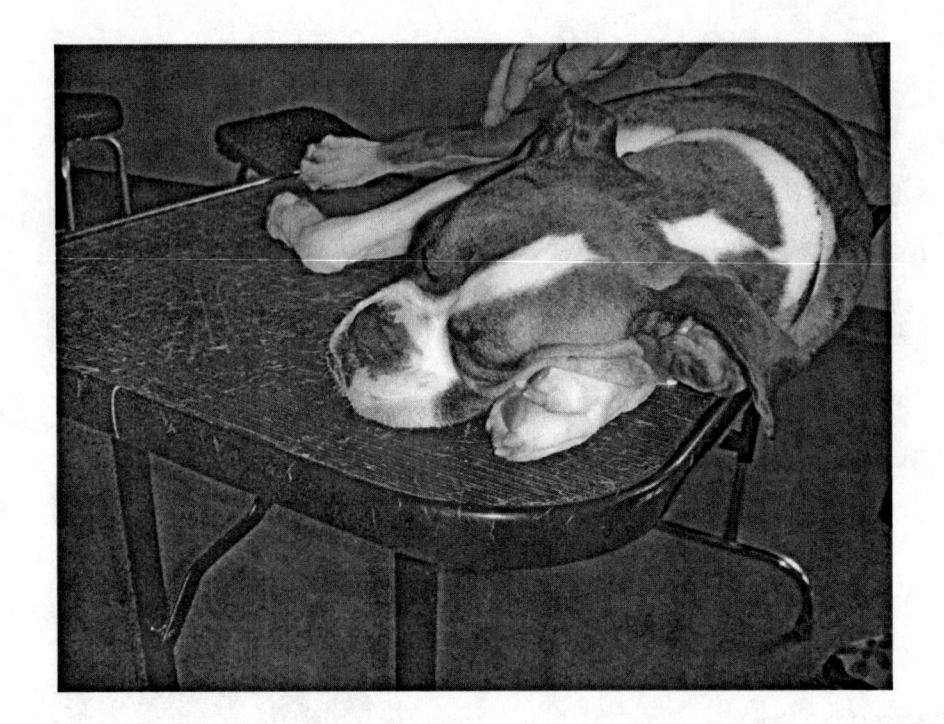

Assessment strokes in series of threes

Assessment strokes help you assess how the dog's body feels to your hands. It's a great way to introduce your dog to your personal touch-print. Work in groups of three strokes in the assessment strokes sequences. Your hands move over specific routes to make sure that you systematically touch, observe and assess your dog's entire body.

Each of the three passes is extremely slow. Each is progressively firmer and more deliberate than the one before. Your hands and fingers move methodically and respectfully into your dog's body space. Your hands and fingers are sensing devices moving over the body, tracing all the bumps, contours and textural qualities.

Your first pass is the most like petting, only with more focus. On this first level, you are observing the texture of the coat, the play of light and shadow, the dirt and dust in the hair and between the toes and how your dog is responding to you. Using light pressure (visualize: presence) this pass says "Thank you for permission to give you a PetMassage. Okay, we're starting now. We are going to spend some very special time together."

The second pass is more connected. Using medium pressure, your touch is more intimate. You observe the textures on and just beneath the skin, and the qualities of the superficial tissues. Notice temperature variations, lumps, and bumps. Notice the general contours and shapes of the body. This pass says, "Let's work together."

Your third pass takes you deeper, where your dog lives. Move slowly. Move deliberately. Move intentionally. Observe the shapes of the muscle groups, the outlines of bones, ligaments and tendons. Notice deeper reflexes and movements such as twitching, tightening or softening of muscles. This pass says, "I'm here to support you."

This is the pattern we will use:

- Dorsal media line: nose to tail
- Right fore leg, starting at the nose moving to the toes
- Left fore leg, starting at the nose moving to the toes
- Right hind leg, starting at the nose moving to the toes
- Left hind leg, starting at the nose moving to the toes
- Ventral media line, underside of the nose to belly

The pace of your strokes sets the mood. The intention in each touch will help you both feel more balanced and connected.

Dorsal media line (top line)
Start at the philtrum, the little divot in the upper lip under the nose, moving up and over the fine hair of the medial line of the muzzle, over the top of the head, over the neck, spine, croup, base of the tail and to the tip of the tail.

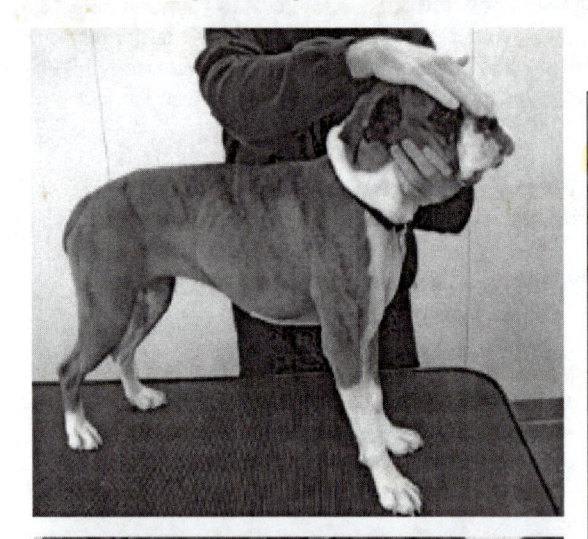

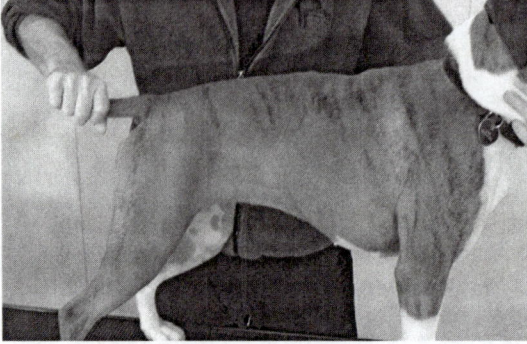

Where the tail has been docked, as you see here, continue each stroke past the tip, acknowledging the rest of the "phantom limb."

In their body/mind memories, they still have the twenty ± vertebrae that would have helped with balance, movement, body-space awareness and communication.

This also applies to amputated limbs and cosmetic surgery, such as clipped ears.

It is not important which order you employ your assessment strokes as long as the entire body is eventually all assessed. Each of the three-stroke assessment sequences begins on the nose, either the philtrum, the sagittal slit, separating the two halves of the nostrils, the slits that open from the lateral sides of the nostrils or the center of the lower lip, below the philtrum.

Stroke in sets of three strokes, moving with the grain, the lay of the hair.

Head, shoulders, forelegs and paws
Apply all three levels of passes, nose to toes. Each stroke begins on the slit on the side of your dog's nose. Continue with the side of the face, over the ear, neck, shoulder, upper arm, elbow, leg, carpus including the dew claw, and toes. Pay special attention to the shoulder blade and point of the shoulder (most proximal end of the humerus). Be sure to include the little toes, the toenails and the pads under the paws.

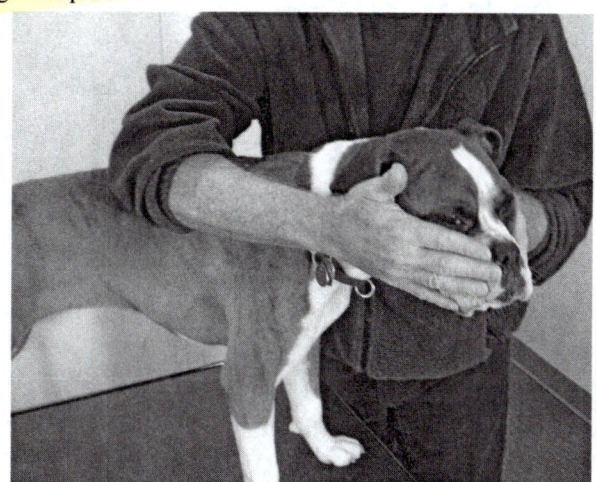

Notice the complexity of the structure of the toes. Dogs have the same number of bones in their toes as do humans in their fingers.

Repeat on the other side: all three levels of passes, light, medium, and deep, from nose to toes. Be sure to include the medial, inner leg, and dogs' residual thumbs, the dewclaws.

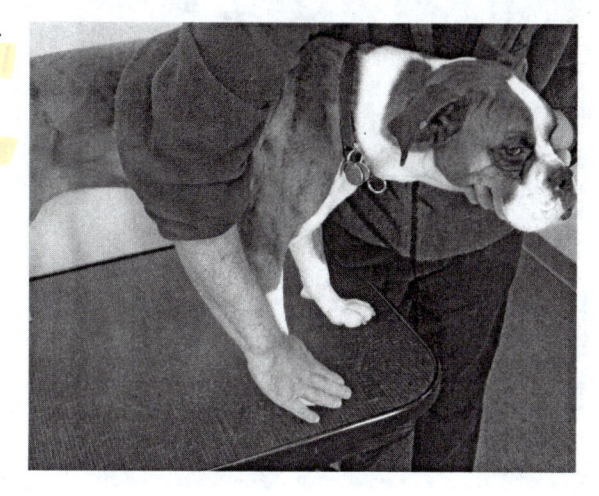

Head, neck, ribs, hips, hind legs and paws

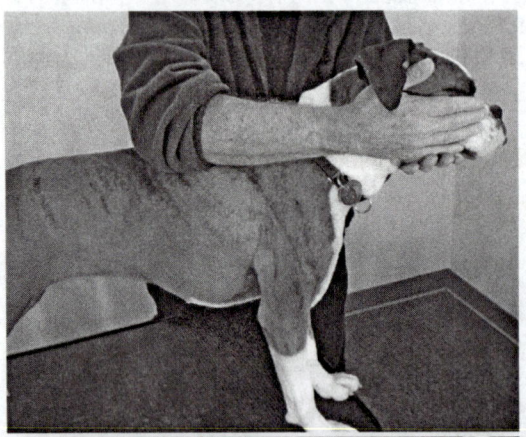

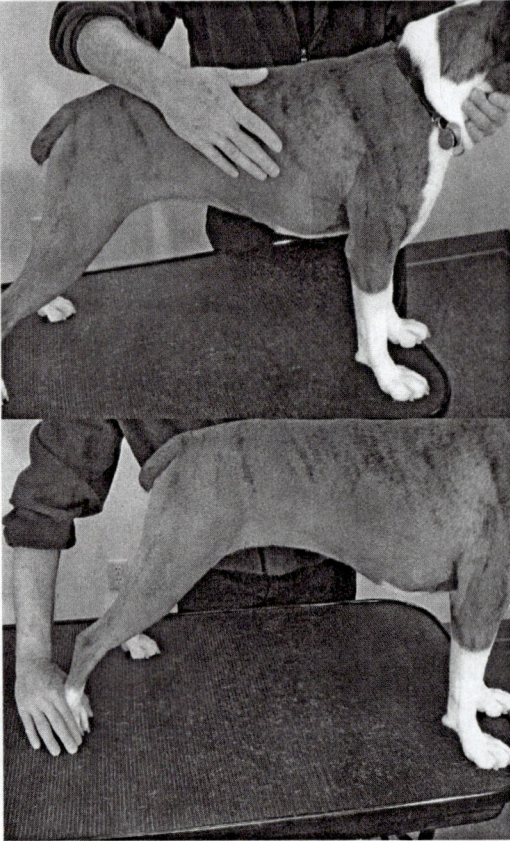

Apply all three levels of passes, nose to toes. Each stroke begins on the slit on the side of your dog's nose. Continue the strokes over the eye, ear, neck, shoulder, ribs flank, hips, hind leg, and toes. Pay special attention to the ribs, hip, large thigh and hamstring muscles.

The wiry tendon that runs over the hock, ankle, to the bottom, the plantar aspect, of the paw is the vulnerable Achilles tendon. Be sure to include the toenails and the pads under the paws.

Other side
Repeat all three levels of passes, nose to toes. Be sure to include the little whirl over the sit bone, the ischial tuberocity, on the caudal side of the pelvis. Notice the rear dewclaws, the stopper pads on the plantar, underside of the paws, toe digits and toenails.

Ventral line

Begin in the middle of the soft underside of your dog's chin. Trace your hand back through the groove formed by his jaw bones, moving over the neck and sternum, to the belly. Three slow, deliberate strokes as above, light, medium, and deep.

Touching alone will only give you a very limited amount of information. Observe with all your senses. Use your nose, your eyes, your ears, your taste, and your sense of spatial comfort.

Incorporate correct breathing, footwork and awareness of your center of balance into each stroke. This is a departure from your previous way of moving, your old holding patterns!

Your mother hand stays in contact with the dog's body. Your active hand is pulled and pushed by your torso.

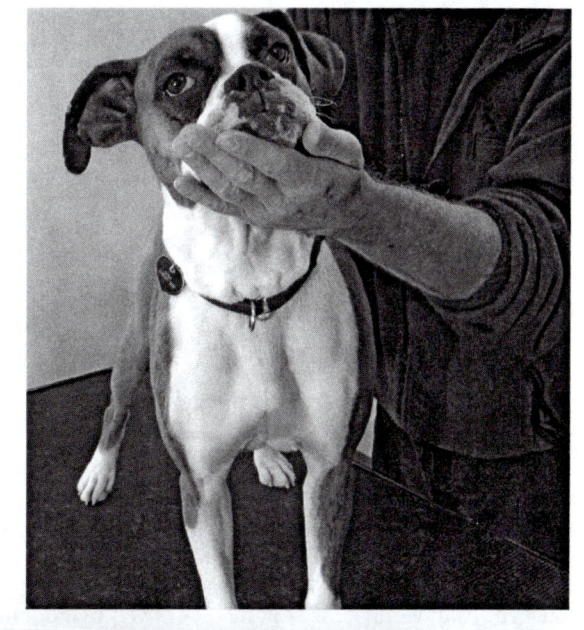

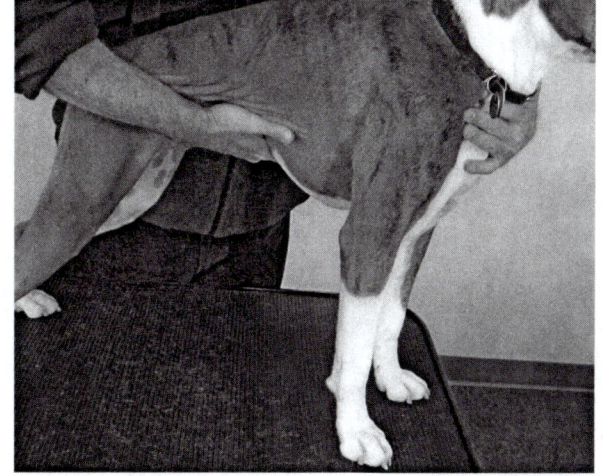

Keep you thumbs up, your elbows down and smile.

Whose assessment

Assessment strokes help you assess how the dog's body feels to your hands. It gives you a systematic way to assess how your dog is responding to your touch.

From your dog's perspective, he gets to evaluate how his body feels when touched. And, while he is at it, he judges you by noticing your responses to him.

Scratching

Scratching, fingernails raking across the body, is the PetMassage movement that is most similar to what dogs do naturally to provide relief from itches and stiffness. It is an intuitive effort to dislodge debris in their skin and hair that is bothersome. Dogs scratch themselves for the same reasons humans do.

Have you observed your dog methodically, raking his hind foot claws across his chin or ear?

It is the same as when we scratch our heads when we are confused, or rub our chins when coming up with a solution to a problem, or massage our temples when we are stressed. It could be a search for a memory. It could be earwax. Both are equally significant, depending on your dog's needs.

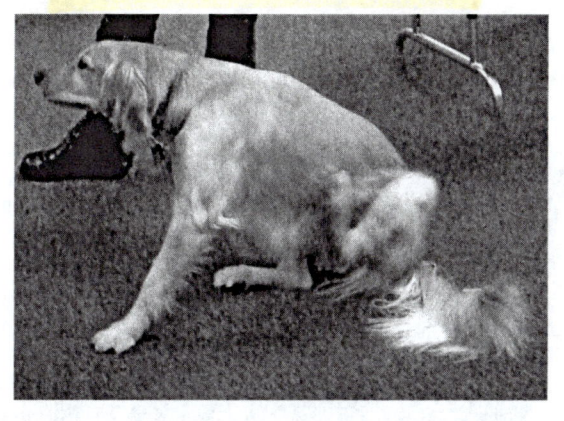

Scratching stimulates cardiovascular, neurologic and lymphatic circulation. Deep, medium, and light pressures of scratch each have different effects.

Scratching on all three levels, and both directions, toward the heart and away from the heart, and over all the major joints is an important part of the Geriatric PetMassage form (see Geriatric PetMassage Session).

Scratching the side of abdomen causes reflexive intermittent leg thumping. You knew that.

Although it may seem counterintuitive, light scratching, barely grazing the surface of the hair, is the most powerful of all three pressures for stimulating your dog's auto-immune system.

Light scratching affects the lymphatic system. Light scratching, brushing your fingernails over the coat toward the heart over lymph nodes supports lymphatic drainage beneath the skin by:

- accelerating filtration from the intercellular spaces into the lymph vessels
- the emptying of the smaller vessels into the larger lymph vessels
- assisting the flow of lymph through the lymph nodes

Medium scratching excites and tonifies the muscles and nerves of the skin, improving venous circulation. These mechanical effects directly enhance capillary circulation as evidenced by a feeling of warmth.

Deep skin scratching penetrates into the tissues. It increases venous blood flow within the skin and the superficial tissues. It stimulates the skin's nerve end-fibers that play an indispensable role in nervous system activity. This explains the remarkable relaxing effect, including decreased muscular tension, elicited by scratching.

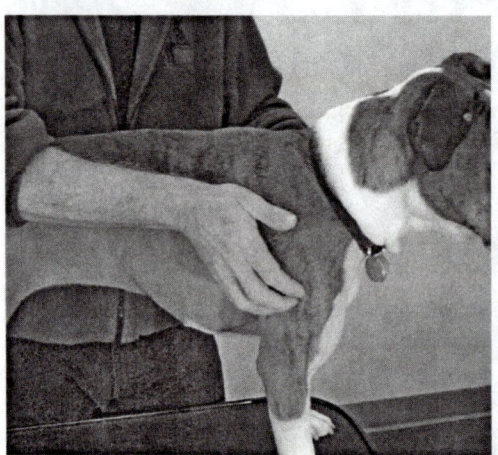

Decreased muscular tension also enhances lung capacity, digestion, bowel movements, blood circulation, lymph drainage and affords for clearer thinking.

Body mechanics
Scratching is stroking with the nails. Your hands are pulled across your dog's body by the movements of your torso. Each scratching gesture involves the use of your entire body. Keep your wrists flexible, your fingers curled, your elbow pointed toward the floor. Long sweeping strokes, running the entire length of the dog's spine are very appreciated. Scratching toward the head is more stimulating than toward the tail. Scratching up the leg is more stimulating than scratching down. Scratching the medial soft coat is more stimulating than scratching the lateral hardier coat.

Repetition

Repetitive scratching and stroking *with* the lay of the coat, creates layers of soothing building to an hypnotic end effect. *Against* the lay of the coat, repetitive stroking and scratching, is highly stimulating.

Rates of movement
Your rates of movement influence how your strokes will be received and integrated. Fast movements stimulate. Slow ones relax. Fast and deep are more stimulating than fast and light. Slow and deep will be more stimulating than slow and light.

Slow strokes, against the lay of the coat are like pushing your fingers through thick summer grass; luxurious, sensual, comfortable, and mildly stimulating. Fast repeated stroking, against the lay of the coat, has caused dogs to get so excited, they bound off the table and race around the room!

- Repetitive stroking with the lay of the coat is relaxing
- Repetitive stroking against the lay of the coat is stimulating
- Slow repetitive strokes moving away from heart, and with the lay of the hair, relax. Direction: cranial to caudal, and proximal to distal.
- Slow strokes moving toward heart, against the lay of the hair are mildly stimulating. Directions: caudal to cranial, ventral to dorsal and distal to proximal
- Slow repetitive strokes, with the lay of the coat calms and relaxes
- Fast repetitive strokes against the lay of the hair are wildly stimulating

Clasped hands

The 2-hands clasped movement moves through the ribs connecting the back to the belly and the belly to the back. It stimulates the circulation and tone of intercostal muscles, diaphragm, and the organs, heart, pericardium, lungs, pancreas, liver and spleen.

Clasped hands provides a dual sensory stimulation. Your hands are maintained in a semi-curled position. Your connection will be through your fingernails and your palms.

Body mechanics

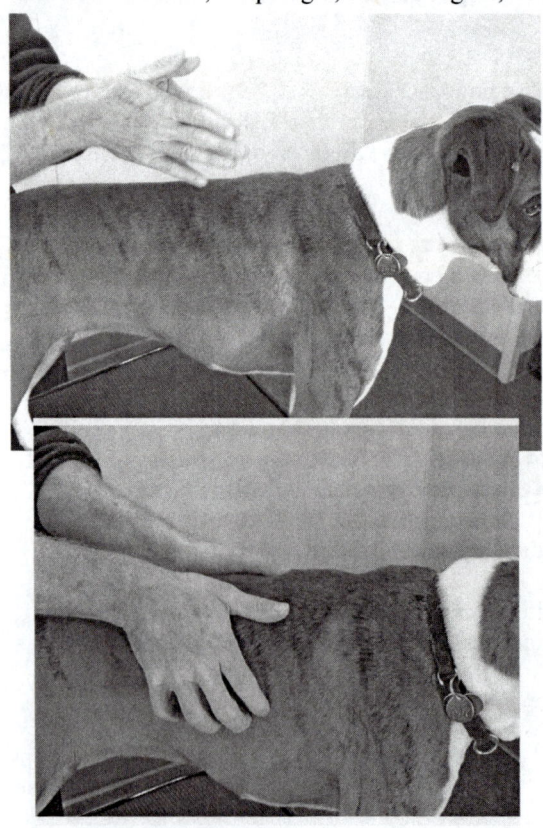

Inhale, bringing your hands together, palms touching. Exhale lowering your fingers onto the spine. As your fingertips touch the topline just caudal to the withers, allow your hands to separate and curl. Scratch with your fingernails, followed by the soothing caress of your palms. Move from the spine to the belly following the grooves between the ribs, the intercostal spaces. When your hands arrive at the belly, allow your fingers to lace.

There is no need to lift the belly. The pattern your fingers make when they weave together will slightly irritate the soft underbelly, the ventral fascia, and causes reflexive muscle spasms. The back muscles tighten, pulling the belly up and away from your hands. Besides stimulating the organs within, this movement also empowers and strengthens the back muscles.

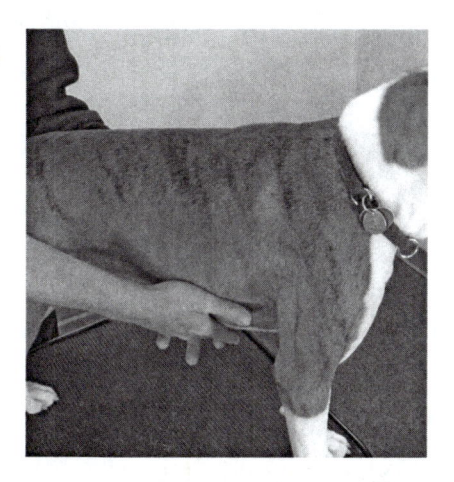

With your hands still laced, step back, inhaling. Allow your weight transfer to pull your palms and fingernails back up, following the same grooves between the ribs to the spine. Keep your arms relaxed yet stationary. Your body moves your arms. Step forward to lower your hands. Step back, pulling them.

Visualize a dog pulling a blanket with his teeth. For him to pull it to one side, he has to turn his body and step back. Make your body push and pull your hands the same way.

Push and pull your hands by shifting your body from foot to foot. Step and turn. Your upper body will follow.

Repeat three or four times flowing down and up, moving from the cranial, forward part, of the ribs to caudal, the back. Experiment with varying depths of pressure.

Usually your dog is standing during his PetMassage. If you do not have to stretch your chest muscles to reach over the dog's back, clasped hands is performed with both hands at the same time.

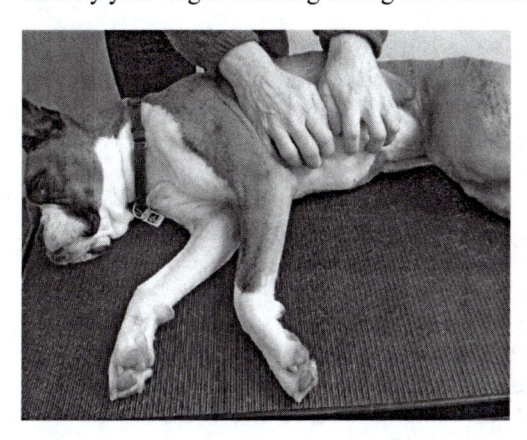

If your dog is on his side or is too high for you to comfortably reach across the topline, work one side at a time. Using one hand or two, your body rocks forward and back, pushing and pulling your hands.

Compression

Compression uses pressure to compact the tissues of the body beneath your hands. Spreading and applying pressure to deeper muscle tissue, it invokes the relaxation response. The motion of pressing and releasing affects the pressure within the vascular system. Compression enhances blood flow and softens the tissues.

Rhythmically alternate one hand with the other. Visualize a cat kneading with its claws. Throat purring is optional, although its vibration has been shown to enhance the effect.

Most compression is applied with the palms, as was your palpation. Press with your palms. Your fingers do no work. They rest and balance the hands. Your focus is now below the skin, pressing the superficial layers of tissue into the deeper ones. Compression is considered deep work. Use compression on the large groups of muscles on the shoulder, back and hips.

Body mechanics
Each press forward begins in your feet. It is the result of your entire body rocking forward. Your body and arm positions are important here. Your arms are relaxed yet partially braced. Your elbows stay quiet, moving neither up nor down. Begin with your hands held in front of you. Your wrists are straight and your palms are directed toward your dog's body. You should be able to visualize a single line running from your forearm over your wrists into your thumbs. It's the same position your arm would be in when you're shaking hands. There are no bracelet creases in the skin on the backs of your wrists.

The rocking motion moves your whole body. Pushing off your rear foot pushes you in toward the dog. Falling back into your rear foot, pulls your body and hands away. Rocking forward, press and roll your hands, heel to fingers. You can rock across the palms from lateral to medial and medial to lateral, as well.

Exhale as you rock forward and into the dog.

Each compression will be the result of transferring your center, from back to forward. There should be virtually no movement or exertion from your arms or shoulders. If you notice that you are engaging your shoulder or pectoral muscles, you are not working from your feet.

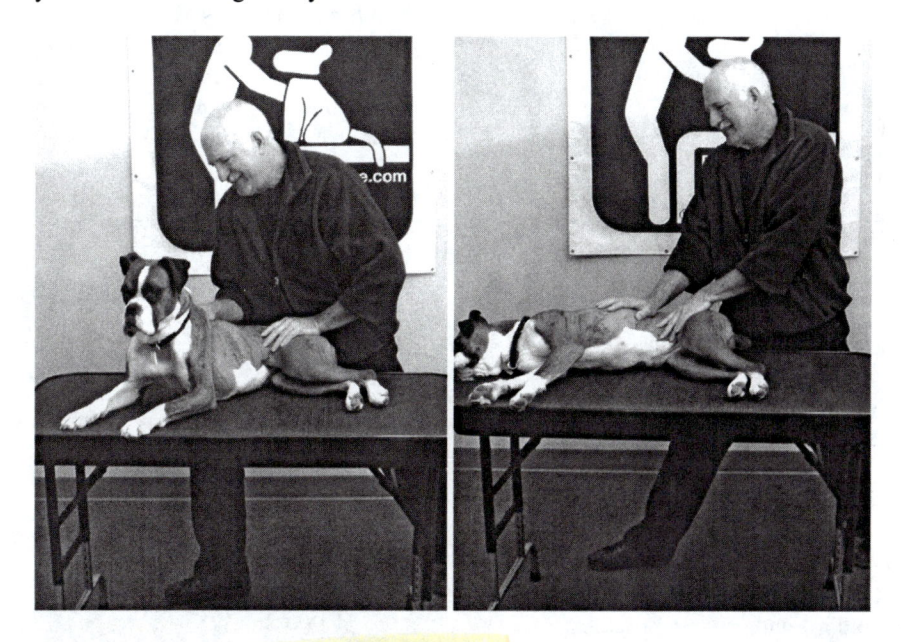

Inhale as you rock back and into the earth.

Transfer your center of gravity from your forward foot into your rear foot. As your center is pulled back, your body pulls your arms and hands with it. Every part of your body, not just your hands, releases your pressure.

When you work starting from your feet, the energy and vitality flow from the bottom, up.

You feel the power and the wisdom of the earth rise up through the soles of your feet and into your core. As you step forward, pressing into the dog's body, exhale out your palms. This is power that your dog knows.

If you were using your shoulders, chest and arms, the energy and intention would be from the top down. Relying on what we think we know limits our choices; especially when compared to what you can do tapping into the wisdom of the earth power. You could be so busy making conscious decisions about pressure, duration and rate of withdrawal, that you could easily miss many significant signals from your dog.

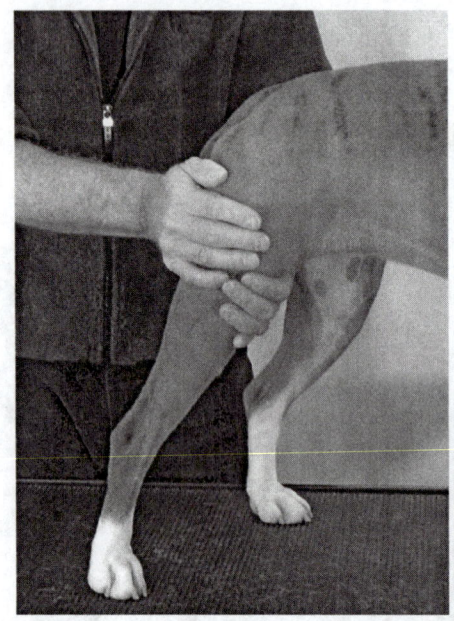

A variant of compression is squeezing the tissues between both palms. This is a greatly supportive movement all the way down the limbs, from shoulder to toes and from hip to toes. It is as if you were giving a series of palmer hand hugs. Coordinate your palmer squeezing movements with your breathing, rather than your footwork.

Exhale as your hands flex toward each other. Inhale as they relax.

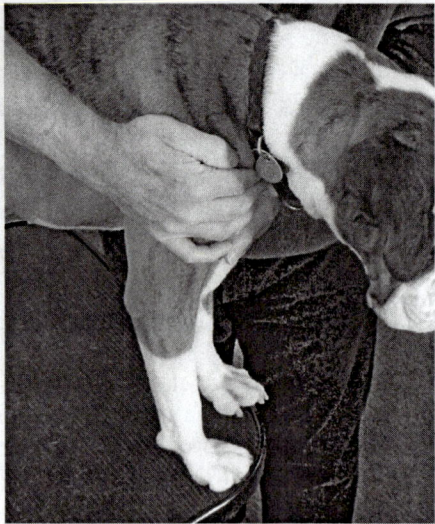

Sweat wrap
Combine compression with still-holding, and you can provide an effective sweat wrap; your hands redirecting the dog's body heat back into and around the muscles. Observe the micro-movements of the tissues against your palms.

Whatever you focus on expands. As you learn to develop patience and pay more attention, your dog, through his experience of your touch, becomes more aware of his own body.

Joint mobilization

Joint mobilization does exactly what it says. It helps increase range of motion within the joint. PetMassage joint mobilization only takes the joint through a very limited range of motion and no further. The movements are smaller, directed inward. This makes the movements more like little course corrections than big stretches that are intended to break down the fibers in the muscle tissue.

Body mechanics
Your hands lightly grasp above the joint and below it, or encase the joint between them. Your Mother hand supports from below or medially. Enter into the technique by rocking forward, exhaling. Allow your body weight to do the little work that has to be done The palm of your active hand moves into the palm of your mother hand sliding the tissues between them up and down, back and forth, from side to side and/or in circular movements. Involve your whole body in each movement. Keep your shoulders and arms stable, with your legs and torso moving your hands. Continue to coordinate your breath with your movements. Circular breathing patterns will reinforce circular hand patterns.

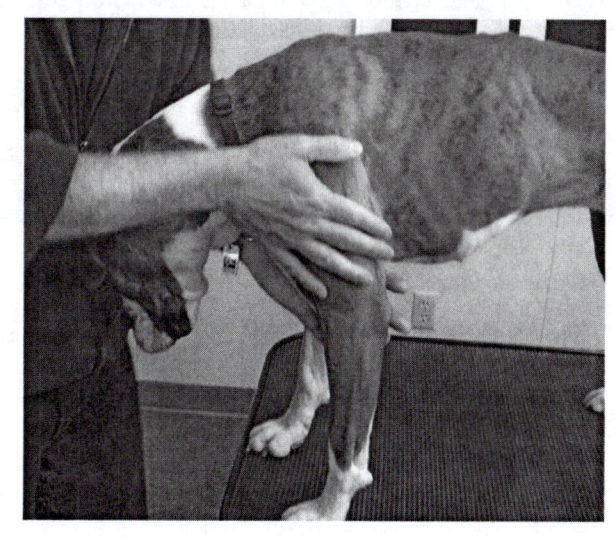

Feel for the quality of movement. Are the tissues gliding easily? Is there a slippery feeling? Do they feel hard, stiff, stuck and restricted? Is there a lot of movement? Is there only a little?

The joints that are good candidates for mobilization are the mandible, the skull and dorsal neck, point of the shoulder, elbow, wrists, knuckles of the paw, the hips, stifles, and hind paws. The rolling motion as the joint is mobilized strengthens tendons and ligament attachment sites.

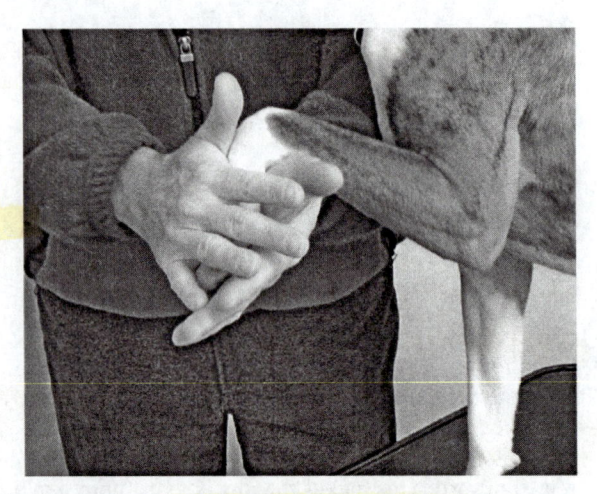

Joint mobilization increases circulation of blood, lymph and all the other fluids within the joint capsules, and in the process revitalizes synovial fluid. Tiny pulsing movements enhance balance to all the fluids, structures and movements within joint capsules.

In joint mobilization, it is important to be able to visualize what is moving about between your hands. If you learn some basic canine anatomy, you will be able to observe with an educated eye and have a more knowledgeable, informed touch. So what is a joint, and why is visualizing it so important?

Synovial Joint

Synovial membrane

Articular cartilage

Fibrous joint capsule

Joint cavity filled with synovial fluid

Ligaments

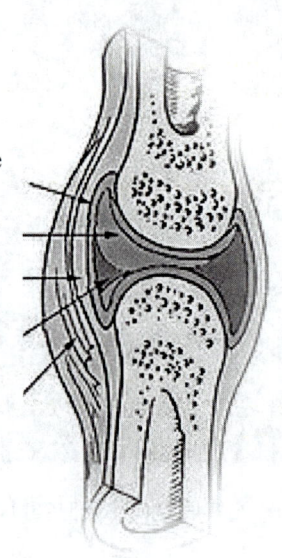

First of all, a joint is the articulation, or juncture of two or more bones. All purposeful movement occurs at joints. Movement happens when the muscles that span a joint contract or relax. That's all that skeletal muscles do. They contract and relax. And, every skeletal muscle spans at least one joint. The ends of muscles, that attach to bones, the tendons, are made of strong inelastic fascia.

The bones that meet have to be directed and limited in their movements; held in place by ligaments, the structures that join bones to bones and act as mechanical reinforcements. Capsular ligaments are part of the joint capsule of synovial joints.

Synovial joints, joints with synovial fluid as a lubricant, are the most common type of joint in the body. Synovial fluid is produced by the joint capsule.

So we have bones that are articulating, communicating with each other, held in place by ligaments and a fibrous joint capsule, moved by the action of muscles, and lubricated by, among other things, synovial fluid.

It is interesting to note that no muscle is an island, that is, no muscle works by itself. All muscles are in groups. They have one of three functions. They are 1) the one initiating the movement, the agonist, or they could be 2) limiting, restricting movement, the antagonist, or 3) supporting the general movement, the synergist.

There are six types of synovial joints. Their names describe their action and/or shape. A hinge joint, for example swings back and forth like a hinge. A ball and socket joint moves like a ball turning in a socket. There are also gliding joints, ellipsoidal joints, saddle joints and the joint between the atlas and axis neck bones (proximal radioulnar joint and distal radioulnar joint).

The factors that influence joint stability are the shape of articular surfaces, capsules and ligament, and muscle tone.

The movements that are possible in synovial joints are:

- Abduction: movement away from the mid-line of the body.
- Adduction: movement towards the mid-line of the body.
- Extension: straightening limbs at a joint.
- Flexion: bending the limbs at a joint.
- Rotation: a circular movement around a fixed point

The movements you will sense within the joints will usually feel more like the bones and tissues are gliding over each other, back and forth and in slight rotation.

Being able to visualize what is happening is especially important when working with dogs that are in rehabilitation, dogs whose joints and muscle attachments are compromised due to obesity, injuries, and dogs with chronic diseases like arthritis or epilepsy. It is also helpful to be able to imagine the body to describe and document what you feel.

The more you know, the better you will be at sensing what is going on within the dog's body. Study basic canine anatomy. Learn more about how the body functions. Study The Canine Anatomy Coloring Book that we use in workshops. [Kainer and McCracken]

Pulling, or tractioning, is a variation on the theme of joint mobilization. It consists of a slow gentle pulling (tractioning) action of the muscles along their axis which causes the bones to pull slightly apart. All skeletal muscles traverse a joint, attaching above and below it. This technique gently stretches and strengthens the tendon-fascia attachment sites.

Pulling or tractioning using successive levels of pressure, nourishes the joint. It helps to balance the functionality of muscles, decreasing muscle tone in overly tight muscles and ligaments and, most importantly, loosening any tissues that cross the joint. This is the mechanical beginning part of positional release.

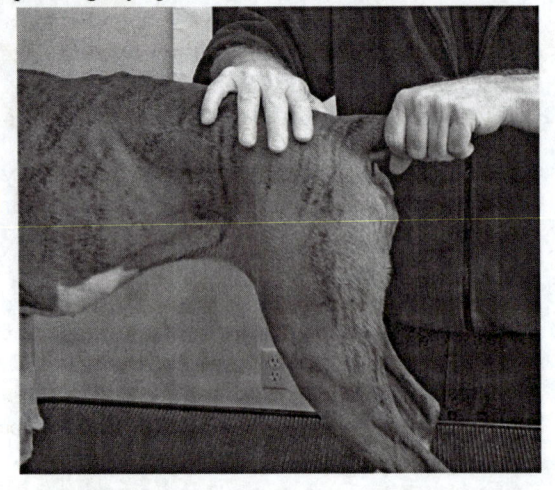

Breathing mechanics
Breathing is as important in joint mobilization as it is in compression. Inhale as your hands move toward you. Exhale as they move away. Inhale as your hands are circling toward you. Exhale as they circle away.

I would caution against using joint mobilization on hocks, (ankles) as this is deep work and hocks, by design, move only in one plane, not in circles.

Also, chiropractic, physical therapy and sports massage joint mobilizations are much more active --and intrusive--taking the joint well beyond its range of comfort and motion; which is not in our PetMassage scope of practice.

Hey, hey. What do you say?

Please notice the vocabulary that we are using. Everything we describe is in terms of what we palpate, what we feel. The qualities of textures and movements we can feel in the coat and the tissues are warm or cool, smooth or rough, tight or loose, resilient or inelastic. Describing them is our focus. We are careful not to name a disease or symptom because naming is diagnosing. And, diagnosing is part of the practice of veterinary medicine, and outside the scope of practice for PetMassage.

So, if you feel swelling, heat and restricted movement in a joint, that is how you would describe what you feel to the dog's guardian or vet. Balanced or imbalanced, are also good terms that may depict what you feel.

There are specific signs and symptoms that we all know for the disease called *arthritis*, which is the diagnostic term for joint inflammation. We are careful not to use the medical term *arthritis*, as that would be diagnosing. There may be other reasons for the presentation of heat and swelling that we do not have the training to know about. Whenever you feel something that causes you concern or is outside your knowledge base, refer your client to her veterinarian or other allied health professional.

During one of our workshops, a student discovered a little black shiny object on her dog's coat. "It's a tick," she declared as she showed it to me. "Give me a tweezers. I'll pull it off."

"Pulling off a tick is a medical procedure," I responded. "It looks as if it's a tick; and yet, I cannot be sure." We left it as we found it. When I returned the dog to her caregiver later that afternoon, I mentioned that her dog might have a tick on her neck. "Oh no," I was told, "That's a growth that we've been keeping an eye on."

What are the first laws of any health care? Do no harm. Support wellness. And, if you are not absolutely positive about what something is and what to do with it, leave it alone.

The pet guardians who bring their dogs to you for PetMassage, especially the ones whose dogs have health issues, hang on every word you say. These clients are often desperate for any information or understanding that might shed light on their dog's condition and treatment. Take extreme care in the vocabulary you use. You are the professional. Your opinion matters. An offhand comment about their precious dog's weight or stance or gait, even in humor, could offend someone who is sensitive and may strike panic into their hearts.

The vocabulary used in the practice of PetMassage is drawn from many sources. These are the life science from which PetMassage was developed:

- Massage therapy
- Occupational therapy
- Animal anatomy
- Animal behavior
- Child Psychology
- Martial arts
- Animal communication
- Parapsychology
- Western Veterinary vocabulary
- Traditional Asian-Chinese Medicine
- Ice skating and ice dancing
- Observation of hardwired body language:
- Medical vocabulary and theory
- Oriental and Eastern Indian philosophy
- Meditation
- Practical experience

Although you cannot legally diagnose, you will have to communicate what you see and feel to other people and in your notes. You will be working with veterinarians and physical therapists. You will also be working with increasingly knowledgeable pet guardians.

The next step is to learn a few more terms that will enhance your practice.

Coming to terms with PetMassage

Anatomical terms are universally accepted. Everyone who needs to communicate clearly can, when they use the correct vocabulary.
This is a short list of definitions of terms for basic movement patterns, directions and landmark root words:

Movements (review):
- Abduction: movement away from the mid-line of the body.
- Adduction: movement towards the mid-line of the body.
- Extension: straightening limbs at a joint.
- Flexion: bending the limbs at a joint.
- Rotation: circular movement around a fixed point

Directions
- Proximal, nearer the center of the body, nearer to the point of reference or to the center of the body than something else is. For example, the elbow is proximal to the hand.
- Distal, away from the point of attachment, describes a body part situated away from a point of attachment or origin. For example, the elbow is distal to the shoulder
- Dorsal, on the upper side of the body
- Ventral, Pertaining to the front or anterior of any structure. The ventral surfaces of the body include the chest, abdomen, shins, palms, and soles
- Medial, along the midline, medial plane, of the body
- Lateral, to the side
- Cauda/Caudad, tail
- Caudal, situated in or extending toward the hind part of the body,
- Cranium, the skull
- Cranial, referring to the involving, or located in the skull
- Rostral, toward the front of the skull (rhymes with nostril)

More pathology than anatomy, you must know these terms, as well:

- Acute, disease or condition that is brief, severe, and quickly comes to a crisis
- Chronic, long-lasting, describes an illness or medical condition that lasts over a long period and sometimes causes a long-term change in the body, repeatedly doing something or behaving compulsively
- Dysplasia, medically unusual growth, unusual development or growth of a part of the body such as an organ, bone, or cell, including the total absence of such a part, as in hip dysplasia
- Sprain refers to ligaments: stretch and/or tear of a ligament, the fibrous band of connective tissue that joins the end of one bone with another. Ligaments stabilize and support the body's joints. For example, ligaments in the knee connect the upper leg with the lower leg, enabling people to walk and run.
- Strain refers to muscles and fascia, an injury of a muscle and/or tendon. Tendons are fibrous cords of tissue that attach muscles to bone.

Kneading

Kneading is the process of bunching up the skin and coat, lifting it off the body and releasing it back onto the body. Kneading, or *petrissage*, is a very powerful way to increase the circulation of blood and the lymphatics within deeper tissues. Along with the coat and skin, kneading stretches the layers of fat under the skin and the sheathes of connective tissue around the muscles.

Kneading, or lifting up, begins slowly and progresses to deeper, firmer lifts.

Body mechanics
Your elbows are held at a fixed, stable angle. As you lower, exhale. Allow the pads of your extended fingers to drop onto the coat. Close your hand, bunching the tissue against your palm.

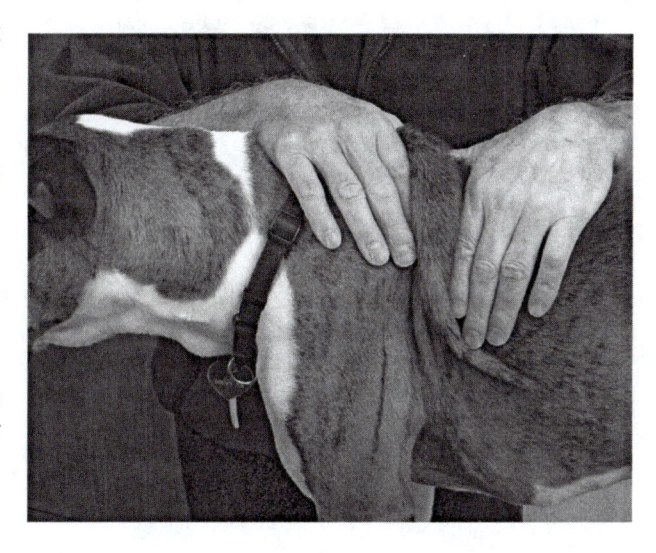

When you inhale your body rises up onto the balls of your feet. Your weight is naturally transferred slightly forward. Your hands are lifted with your body.

Rock backward, exhaling. Release the skin back onto the body, and collect another palmful. Shift your weight forward and back. Make sure that your body does the work, not your arms and shoulders. Your fingers press and release against your palms squeezing, lifting and dropping the coat.

Use your whole body. When you inhale and draw the energy into you tighten all the sphincter muscles in your body. Purse your mouth, pull your shoulder blades together, and flex the muscles of your pelvic floor. Yes, Kegels are part of PetMassage body mechanics.

As you exhale, release your grip. Your whole body relaxes as you fall back into your rear foot.

The process of kneading is a lot of fun to do. Alternate your hands; picking up with one as you release with the other. Work up and down the spine. Knead your way over the shoulders and withers, and up and down the neck. Synchronize your breathing with your dominant hand.

Having difficulty coordinating your breathing? Not to worry. This is also a skill that will come naturally. The body mechanics described here may be a new way for you to use your body. It may feel awkward at first. Anything one tries for the first time feels foreign and difficult. The second time will be a bit easier. The third, easier still. Soon, your muscles will remember how they are supposed to work without your mental interference. This is an exercise in *muscle memory*.

Since the body mechanics we teach are not immediately comfortable, many students of PetMassage decide to continue moving as they always have. These are the students who do not progress beyond where they started. Practice the breathing and rocking and footwork until they are second nature. Later, when we include *positional release* and *follow-on*, you will already be incorporating the correct muscle memory.

Play with these variations to the basic techniques of compression and kneading.

- Experiment with observing the different responses your dog gives you at different depths, directions, and rates of movement.
- Experiment with holding your breath, standing on one foot, sitting on a stool, or sitting on the floor.

Skin rolling

Skin rolling is a variation of kneading. It allows a release in the superficial restrictions between the skin and underlying tissue. It may be necessary to repeat skin rolling a few times over the same area in order to release any long term adhesions.

Skin rolling increases blood flow through the tissues and supports the elastin, the chemical that helps the skin to be resilient, supple, and well, elastic.

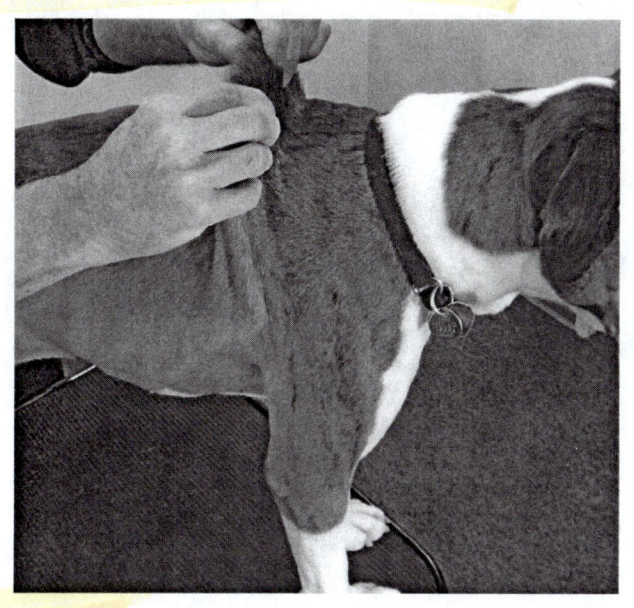

Body mechanics
At the top of your stretch, inhale as you lift your knuckles back toward your nose. Your fingertips draw up across your palms. The skin you are grasping is rolled and stretched between them. Exhale as you release your grip on the

tissues. Do not just let go of the skin and coat, allowing them to snap back. That would be interpreted as disregarding the tissues and the stockpile of memories stored in them. It might feel as if they no longer held any value to you, once you were done with them. Allow them to slip out of your palms slowly and gradually.

As your inhale buoys your body up, your hands come with you. Your exhale drops your body back into your heels, lowering your hands.

Cross skin-rolling is the same movement moving the tissues across the spine, laterally, from side to side. Pick up and pull the skin with one hand while pushing an adjacent patch of skin with the other hand. Cross-skin rolling produces dynamic stimulation to the entire spinal apparatus.

As your hands create stronger and deeper folds, curves and patterns in the coat, you will see how much more flexibility he is developing. Flexibility indicates release of tension and increased circulation.

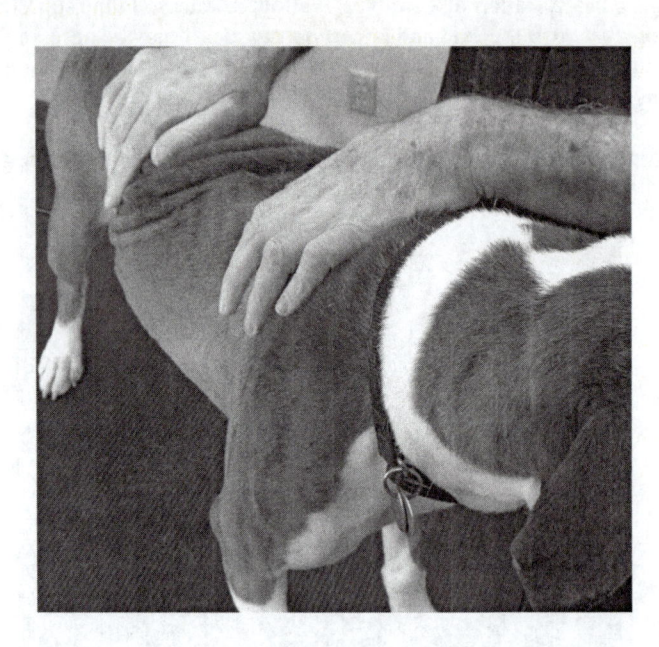

I'll have that with a twist

This simple technique takes skin rolling to the next level. Skin rolling with a twist at the top enhances the stretching and helps to realign the fibers in the connective tissue that contain the muscles.

Twisted skin rolling can be very effective with the lightest of pressures. Experiment on your face, cheeks and around your eyes, lightly plucking the skin by snapping your fingertips. It is stimulating. It is relaxing. It's addictive!

Skin rolling with a twist is effective over recently healed injuries, where adhesions and scarring had developed, on the top of the head, on the neck under the ears, on the hip joint, and on the digits of the paws.

Body mechanics
As your knuckles rise, move your elbow either laterally, to the side or medially, toward the middle of your body. Release the tissues back onto the body gently.

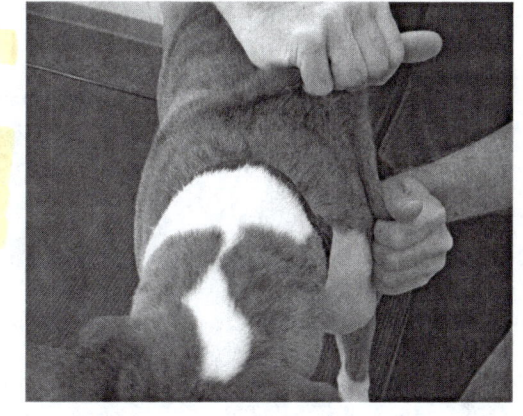

For smaller areas, or parts of the dog that are held tight to the body, use just your thumb and fingertips. The plucking motion with a twist is the same as snapping your fingers against the coat.

Practice these techniques around the sides of the dog's head, neck and hip, and can be combined with frictioning and joint mobilization.

Muscle squeezing

This a term for literally squeezing or compressing the dog's muscles between the palm of the hand and your fingers. Pressure is directed slightly upwards. This should be done slowly at the beginning of the treatment. Pressure will increase with each compression - within your dog's pain tolerance.

Body mechanics
The key to squeezing muscles is to incorporate your whole body in to the movement. When your hands squeeze, everything tightens. You inhale, squeezing your heart with your lungs, your muscles in your forearms tighten, your face tightens, your gluteals tighten.

Your release, is also coordinated with your breathing. As you exhale, your entire body exhales, relaxes and releases.

Experiment with your dog. Notice the difference in his responses when you squeeze and release holding your breath and when you coordinate your breathing with your hands. Notice the difference in his response comparing squeezing with all your muscles and just with your fingers.

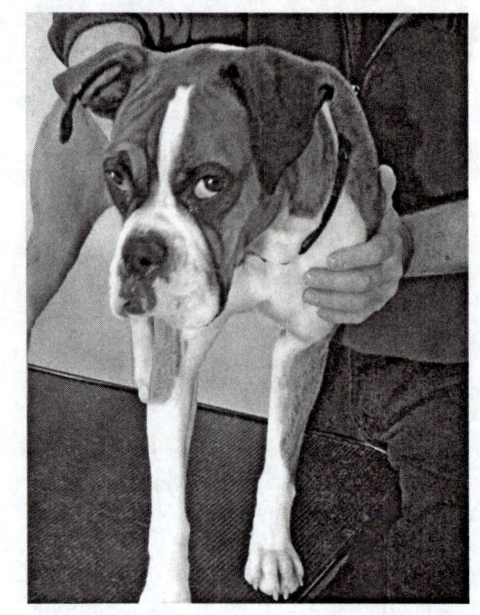

Frictioning

Frictioning is used to help break down connective tissue, or adhesions, found in the fascia. These could be the result of injury or inflammation. To prevent injury and soften tight tissues and get them to participate, it is necessary to warm them. Frictioning will have significant roles in sports and geriatric PetMassage.

Frictioning is a rapid circular or back and forth motion of your hands over the surface of your dog's body. Frictioning creates heat; which is what we want. You can use your thumbs, fingers or palms in small back and forth movements to friction across, perpendicular to the direction of, the muscles. Frictioning moves across the surface of the tissues and also pulls the tissues beneath the skin with it. Sliding the superficial tissues across deeper structures creates deeper heat.

Greater pressure or faster movement will induce more heat, and more circulation.

A good gauge for when the tissues have begun to warm is that you feel warmth in your palms.

Frictioning is an efficient way to warm the tissues prior to kneading or skin rolling. For example, to warm the foreleg, friction by placing your palms on both sides of the leg and rub them vigorously laterally, across the contour of the muscles, starting proximally and moving down to the paws.

Body mechanics
Use your body to move your hands, not your arms and shoulders. Transferring your weight from foot to foot, will turn your hips. Your body should look like it is dancing a very fast "twist." Visualize your body rotating back and forth like a rapidly twisted potted palm tree.

Coordinating your breathing with your footwork is not possible with frictioning. It's important to continue breathing, though. If you do run out of breath, pause, and regroup by focusing on your breathing.

Continue to keep your hands on the dog. In the vocabulary of canine body language, when the hands disengage, the dog's session is over.

Frictioning the hip

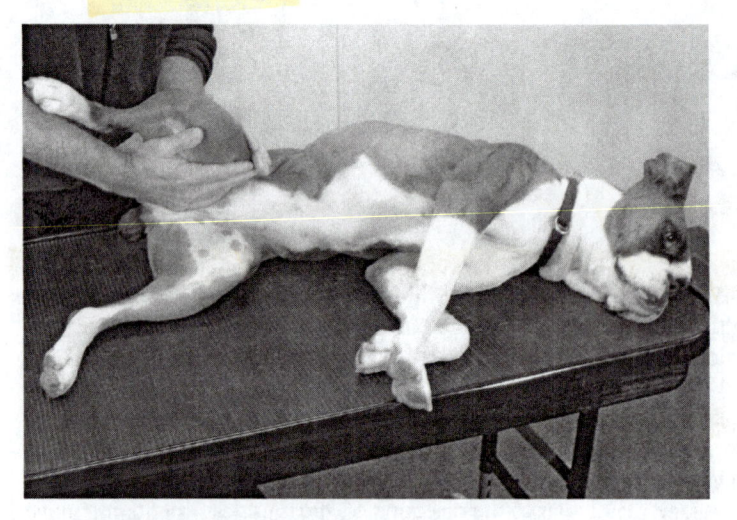

Frictioning the shoulder

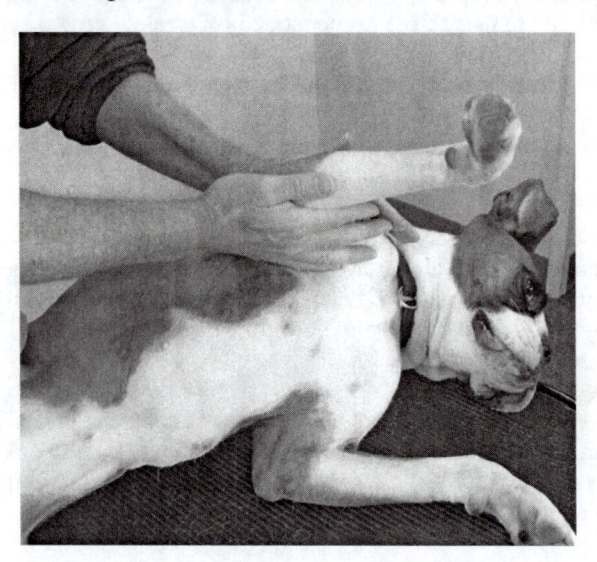

Tapotement -- percussive strokes

Tapotement, or tapping, is a collection of brief, repetitive strikes made with the hand or parts of the hand. These have a stimulating, compressive effect to the skin and tissue. Tapotement has several applications, the most popular being part of pre-event warm up before physical activities. Tapotement reflexively tones the muscles which makes an ideal technique during conditioning and sport training.

Fingertip tapotement is usually described as light tapping with the fingertips. This stimulates tight muscles and decreases fatigue. It enhances awareness and stimulates circulation of blood vessels closest to the surface of the body.

While this technique works well on a human face to tighten skin, very soft tapping can be annoying to a dog. Whenever you tap on your dog, tap with authority. Tapping is done from the wrist. Your palms and fingers are always loose, relaxed and flexible.

Heavy rain drops
Heavy rain drops is a strong, more stimulating tapping with the fingertips. The full weight of your hand and fingers flops forward as you allow the pads of your fingertips to rain down onto the surface as heavy rain drops.

Body mechanics
Use one hand at a time or alternate hands. Use this technique on the head, over the shoulders, the spine and hips. Your palms are loose, relaxed and flexible. Your fingers are relaxed and spread slightly apart. Tap with your movement coming from your forearm and wrist. Make the raindrops heavy!

Contraindication
All types of percussion carry the contraindication that you **never administer percussion over the kidneys** which are located on both sides of the spine just behind, or caudal to, the ribcage. This is a very sensitive area that is highly vulnerable to injury.

Fingertip tapping the spine:
fingers are spread, relaxed and flexible. Movement originates in the wrist.

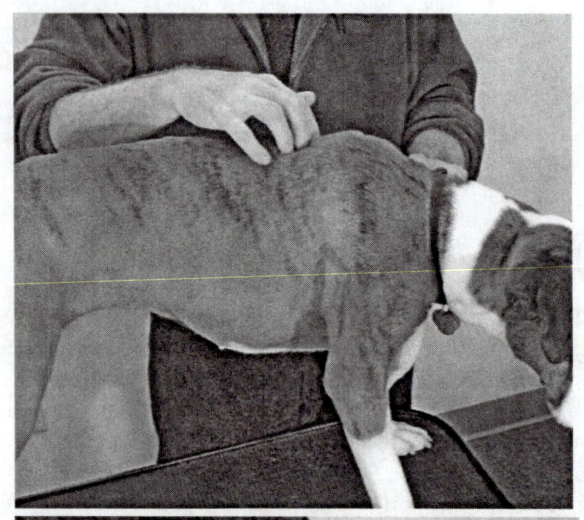

Heavy rain drops on the shoulder: strike with the pads on the tips of your fingers, not with your nails.

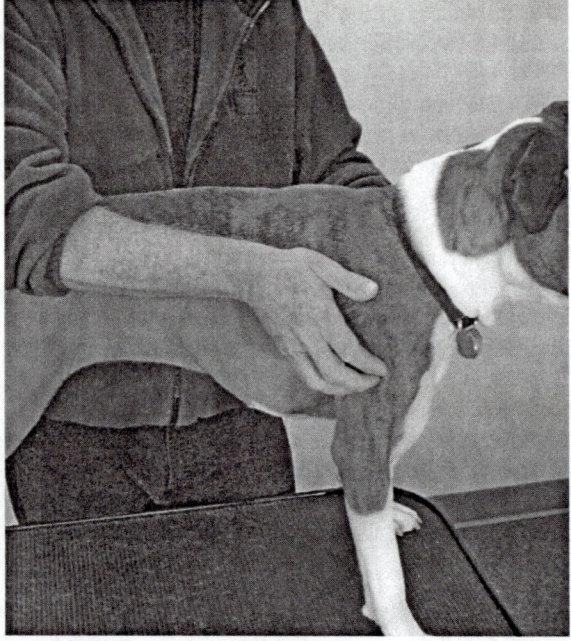

Finger flicking

Light to heavy finger flicking, is done with the ulnar border (baby finger side) of your little finger. Your hands are held closed, as loose fists with your knuckles purposefully spread apart. At impact, the spread fingers bounce into each other, softening the blow and multiplying the numbers of vibrations.

Finger flicking is
- extremely useful for athletes before an event
- blood is drawn to the surface; circulation is improved
- induces muscle tone and strengthens muscles since it stimulates muscles to contract
- over the abdomen flicking increases peristalsis, thereby aiding conditions such as constipation

Body mechanics
Your palms and fingers are loose, relaxed and flexible. Always finger flicking with a soft wrist action. If your wrist is stiff, or your fingers are tight, flicking could have the harming effect of a karate chop.

Incorporate your whole body in each flick. The fingers cannot bounce until the body transfers its inertia into them. Continue to breathe.

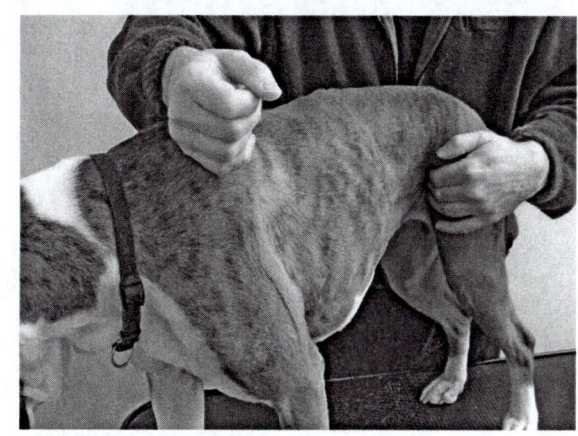

Slapping

Open hand percussing is called slapping. Slapping stimulates the tissues and increases blood flow. It too is used as part of a sports warm up PetMassage. Apply slapping over the large muscles of the shoulder, the ribs, and the top on the skull. Repetitive gentle slapping on the foreface, helps the cerebral sinus fluid balance and encourages the fluids in the superficial sinuses to drain.

Body mechanics
While the slap is applied with the active hand, make sure that you are maintaining contact with your supporting Mother hand. When using the open hand slap, always remember to keep your wrist flexible. If your wrist is stiff, or if you are slapping from a distance, it could feel like punishment and have the harming effect of hitting.

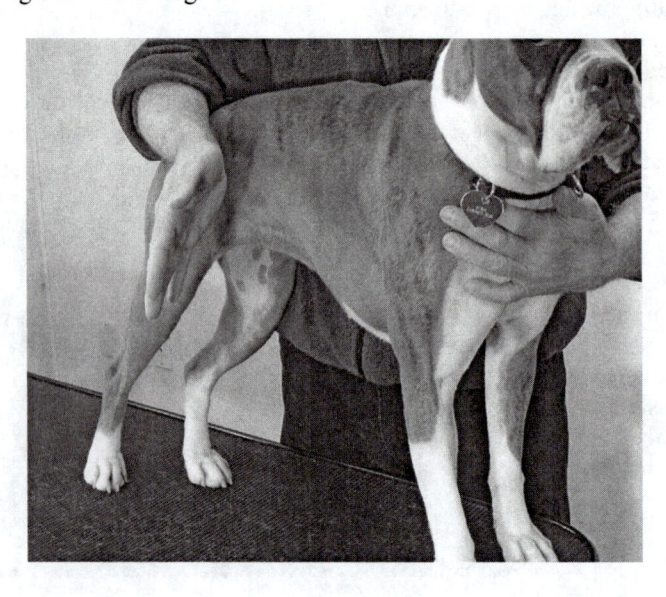

Cupping

Most of our dogs live indoors and breathe in whatever is in the carpets. When outdoors, they breathe whatever is closest to the ground: chemical sprays, fertilizers, toxic fumes from cars, and general pollution residue. All this stuff gets stuck in the lungs, lodged in the surfaces lining the lungs. In time, this debris can compromise the exchange of Oxygen for CO_2 during normal breathing. When dogs do not get enough exercise or are retaining too much phlegm in their lungs, heavy tapotement, or cupping, can dramatically enhance their quality of life. Cupping creates vibrations that resonate deep into the tissues within the ribcage. It shakes the surfaces, dislodging phlegm and toxins.

Cupping makes a hollow sound, compared to the flat, slapping of the open hand or the thin whacking of the finger flick. The sound should be like a horse trotting.

Body mechanics

Cupping is the most powerful of the percussive techniques. Cupping is performed *ONLY* on the ribcage. It is applied with force. Whack the sides of your dog's ribs and over the sternum. Continue until your dog coughs, or expectorates. This could take as long as ten to fifteen seconds of powerful cupping. Include cupping in every PetMassage session.

Cupping, uses the concave surface of the palm, fingers and thumb held together firmly to form a cup. Make a cup with your hand by holding your palm facing up, supine, and pressing your fingers tightly together, as if you were holding water in them. Your fingers are held in this fixed rigid position, however, your wrist is flexible. When you transfer your weight from one foot to the other, and turn your body, your arm is propelled toward your dog's ribcage. Your wrist flips your cupped hand against your dog's ribcage like the tip of a bullwhip.

Cupping is performed *ONLY* on the ribcage.
Cupping is performed *ONLY* on the ribcage.
Cupping is performed *ONLY* on the ribcage.

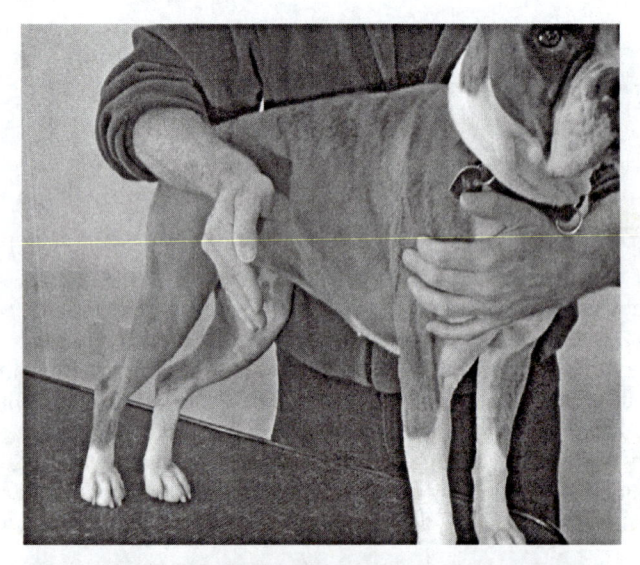

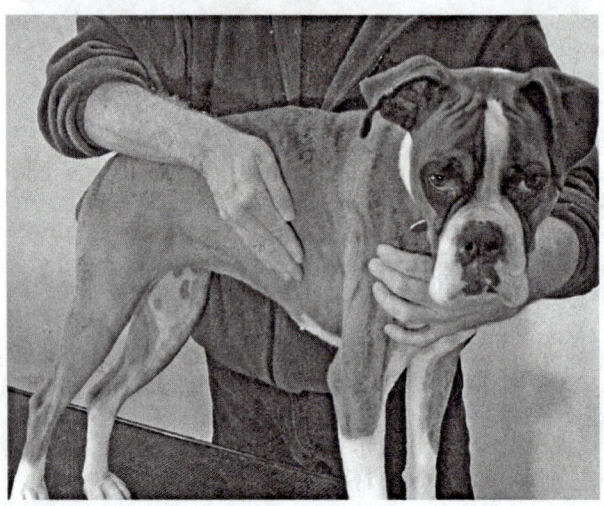

Thymus thump

You may have noticed the handlers at agility competitions and dog shows give their dogs congratulatory pats on the chest after their events. The dogs jump up after their performances, presenting their chests for their reward-thumps. It feels natural, as the handler, to pat them on the chest. The dogs obviously enjoy it.

Thymus thumping is a rapid volley of two or three cupping percussions over the area of the thymus gland, which is located just beneath the top of the sternum in the dog's chest. It is used at the completion of every PetMassage. The Thymus thump offers a very interesting type of stimulation to a very special gland.

The stimulation is deep, as described in cupping. When the cupping is applied over the whorl of hair over the upper part of the sternum, the sound is more like a "thump." The vibration it creates resonates deep into the chest into the thymus gland. This gland is sensitive. It is highly responsive to percussion. Thump your own chest three of four times. You'll feel a bubbling effervescence around your heart.

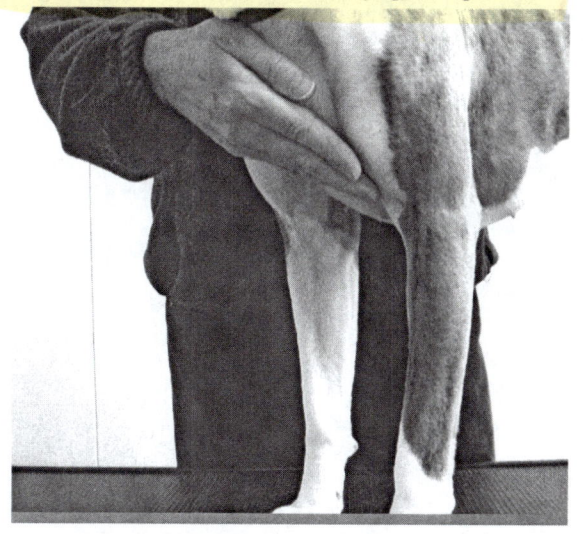

Very little is scientifically known or accepted as general knowledge about this gland. It can be measured and appears to shrivel when the body is fighting disease or dies. For many years it was medically discounted and considered to be folklore since on cadavers, there was nothing left to measure. The thymus is largest during high growth periods and youth. It becomes smaller as we age. The size, and therefore its capacity of whatever it does, is related to vitality, health, and wellness.

John Diamond, MD, writing in his *Notes on the Spiritual Basis of Therapy*, places the functions of the thymus gland in a spiritual context. He maintains that the "*thymus* activity ... involves a putting out from the heart, the spirit rising up to the Divine and going out to other people, the spirit of personal love and concern for all objects on the earth, and of course, deeper than this, an aspiration to be reunited with the Divine. Love for our fellow man and for God are the deep properties that keep the *thymus gland* active... (The) *thymus* activity is the controller of the life force."

The word thymus, was the Greek equivalent to the Traditional Chinese Medicine, Chi. It was derived from the Greek *thymos* which is untranslatable into modern terms; but denotes the concepts of life force, soul, and feeling or sensibility. Thymos originally referred to the breath. "It was the stuff of consciousness, the spirit, the breath-soul, upon which depended on a man's energy and courage." [Diamond]

Thumping the area over the thymus gland stimulates all good feelings, and encourages your dog's intention to maintain mind, body, spirit, health and wellness.

It's a great way to express the wishes, "thank you" and "have a good life."

Shaking

Shaking affects the sensory nerves in the muscles and joints.

It reduces muscle tightness and reflexively relaxes the dog. Shaking, aka, jostling, increases flexibility in muscle tissue and ROM, range of motion in a joint. Applying what we know about fascia, it also increases the ROE, range of emotion. Shaking breaks up and releases mind-body restrictions held within the joint. Shaking can be performed as a continuation of rocking, joint mobilization or positional release.

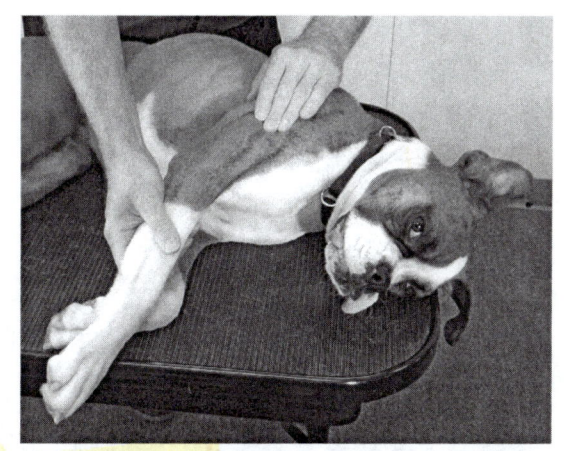

Body mechanics
For tightly restricted muscles, grasp the belly of the muscle, and shake it gently from side to side. For tight and restricted joints, use indirect shaking. Loosely hold the limb proximal to and close to the joint you are shaking. Always shake from the body side, not from the foot. *The limb must be supported.* Uncontrolled wobbly movements can injure the joints and ligaments. As it is shaken, the weight of the limb flops it back and forth, stretching the ligaments and tendon attachments.

Be cautious in the amount and vigorousness that you shake your dog. Stay very gentle and mindful during shaking, watching closely how your dog is responding. The momentum of the limb can hyper-extend the tendons and ligaments. It takes very little to create soreness and possible injury. Work at an even rhythm. Begin slowly with small movements, increasing the motion as the tissues become flexible. Just a few shakes can stretch the tissues. See for yourself by flopping your wrists up and down.

Rocking

In rocking, the body is rocked back and forth in rhythmic patterns. Rocking also reflexively relaxes tight muscles. It has many benefits, and is often used to treat dogs with tight muscles, joint problems, and osteoarthritis.

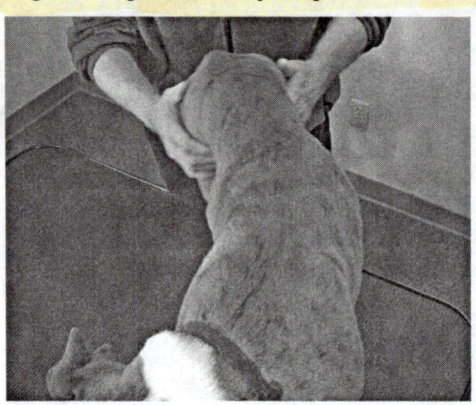

Rocking affects the dog, inside and out. Its movement supports the peristaltic action of the gut to support digestion. It reminds the spine of its possible flexibility by initiating greater movement and frees the central nervous system by breaking down restrictions.

Rocking balances fluids in the inner ear, thereby enhancing proprioception, the awareness of the orientation of one's limbs in space. It helps dogs maintain balance, supports development of bone density as part of a weight bearing exercise when the dog is standing, and enhances the dog's Limbic System, their emotional brain when he is side-lying.

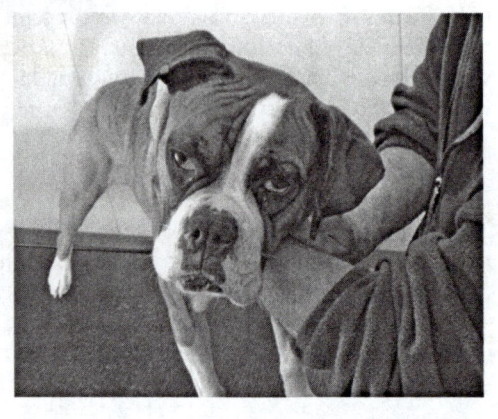

Standing dog
Rocking your dog is fun. With your dog in a standing or sitting position, lightly hold both sides of his/her head, neck, body, or pelvis between your hands and rock your body from side to side, tossing it back and forth from hand to hand.

Body mechanics
Only minimally do you incorporate your shoulders and pectoral muscles into the rocking movement. Your body moves when you shift your weight from one foot to the other. Your arms move when your body turns. Each time your weight is over one foot, it plants that foot onto the ground, grounding yourself. When transferring your weight to your other foot, you draw the energy of the earth up into your body. That energy is supporting your dog from the insides of your palms. You are employing the power of the whole planet. You twist, your dog rocks, the fascia rolls, and the earth moves!

Side-lying dog
When your dog is side-lying rocking helps her organs within her body to nestle into each other. It relaxes the muscle groups that are normally used for maintaining posture. It assists the movement and reorientation of all the fluids within the tissues.

Body mechanics
Stand with your feet shoulder width apart. One of your feet is closer to the dog (the one you will be stepping into when you rock forward). Place both palms on your dog's body and, with your spine straight, your wrists soft and flexible, and your elbows locked, rock her body forward and back, forward and back.

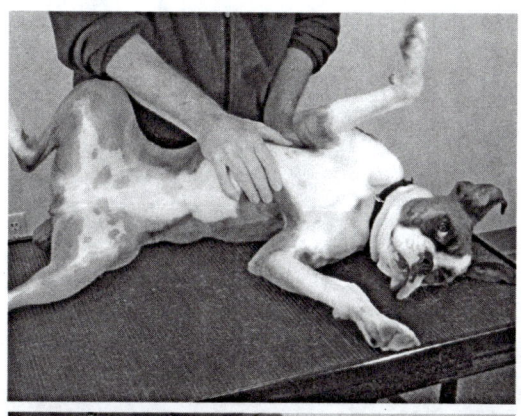

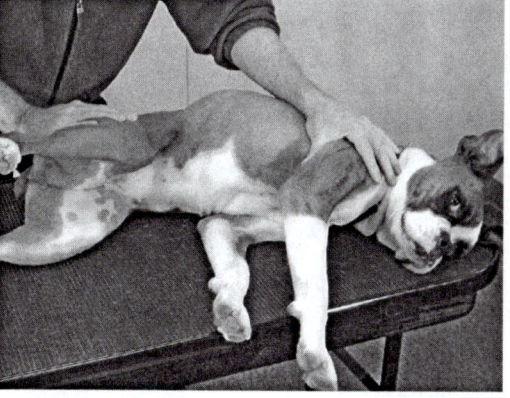

Your propulsion comes as you transfer your weight from one foot to the other. Step forward, pushing, and fall back, releasing.

Rocking doesn't have to be only back and forth. Move in whatever patterns are the most effective: side to side, front to back, ovals and figure eights.

Experiment to discover the most effective rates of rocking. Your dog's body will let you know that you are moving at optimum speed by relaxing into the movement. Continue to breathe normally. There is a tendency, partly because rocking is such a powerful modality, for the student to hold her breath.

Holding patterns

A holding pattern is the unconscious way the body holds itself and uses its muscles. It is the habitual way it interprets and moves about in its surroundings. A holding pattern could be the posture your dog assumes when he eats out of his bowl. It could be the posture your dog assumes when he sleeps. It could be his unique style of walking or trotting.

It could be his response to the question, "Where's that squirrel?"

When people and dogs are experiencing a traumatic event, something that is highly stimulating (in a good way) or that threatens the sense of safety, we automatically gasp and catch our breath. This is a naturally protective reflex that locks the episode and our reaction to it in our bodies. This could be helpful, for example, if you've burned your hand on a hot stove. The memories of your discomfort and the cause of it lock in. This reflex can be detrimental, too.

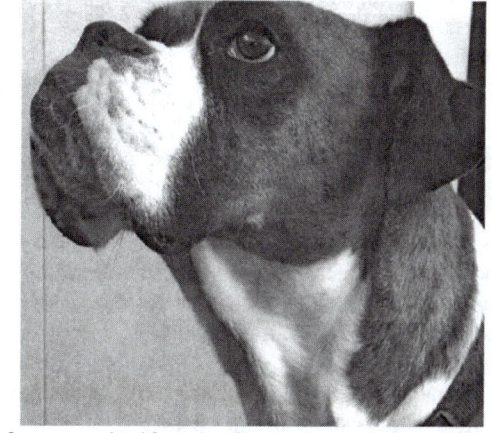

Perhaps your dog lives with other dogs and has discovered that he is most comfortable in the role of follower. He maintains his choice of pack status by sending a consistent body language signal that indicates he is submissive and non-threatening. He carries his chin low to the ground. His shoulder and neck musculature strain and stretch to support his posture of always looking up toward a superior power. Soon his conformation changes to support this posture. He is holding the patterns of developed muscle tone, of follower, and of submissive. His patterns are emotional, physical and psycho-social.

One of the main tenets of PetMassage is that each dog develops its own uniquely individualistic ways of posturing and moving to support its *perception* of safety and wellness. Another is there is memory of everything the dog has ever experienced locked within the tissues of his body.

A dog's habitual way of moving can begin any time during his life. It may start as a simple shifting of weight to relieve pain. A limp might have been a way to compensate for weakness of a limb after an injury or surgery. Just as repetitions of movement patterns soon become second nature, many dogs continue to limp long after their legs have healed.

The body remembers things that feel good; and things that are unpleasant. It remembers how others respond to it when it assumes various postures. Dogs could notice that when they limp they get extra attention. This perk is an incentive to continue the behavior.

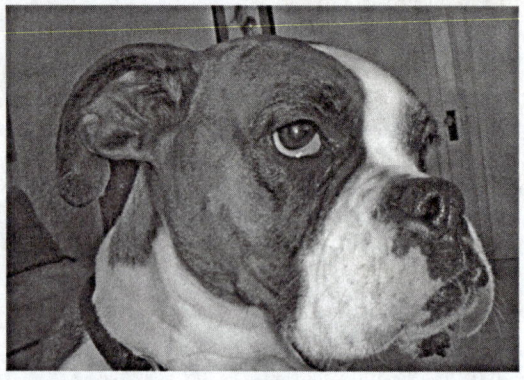

Actually, like humans, the dog's body retains the memory of the emotional response to the event, rather than the specific event. Whether the source is an accident, a surgery, a result of overtraining, or even the grieving of a lost family member, it is their spontaneous emotional responses that determine how they will choose to move their bodies.

The habits that they form, their habitual patterns of movement and emotional responses, are their holding patterns.

Holding patterns are developed, stored in each of the cells of the body fascia. For the body fascia as a whole to function, each cell must retain its own integrity while maintaining a relationship with the rest of the body. The interconnected memories of emotions held within the cells and their adjacent tissues throughout the body create the holding patterns.

In addition to retaining every experience in this lifetime as cellular memory, cells hold all the genetic information. Think of it as all of the cultural memories inherited from previous generations. There are the breed characteristics and, more specifically, breed line characteristics. German shepherds, for example, have certain traits. You see a German shepherd and you immediately recognize the breed and can make some fairly accurate assumptions about temperament, movement, intelligence, health concerns and longevity. This is the breed memory. Within the greater German Shepherd population, some of the breed lines have developed weak hips, or poor eyesight. These are also aspects of memory encoded their bodies.

The responses you can observe in dogs during and after their PetMassage are adjustments to their holding patterns. You may see more vitality and spring in the gait. A freaked-out dog might experience an Alpha state. There will be variations in the sheen of the coat. You may see that your dog is beginning to exhibit signs and symptoms of a healing crisis. [Goldstein]

Deeply rooted memories are so deep that not even the dog knows they are there, even when they have been stimulated. The tiny course corrections are deeply subconscious. Cellular. Shifts on these levels initiate micro-variations, chemical reactions, and twitches of enlightened awareness in deeper tissues and their locked in long-term memories. Once initiated, they have the potential to surface affecting the superficial tissues and more current physical and emotional conditions.

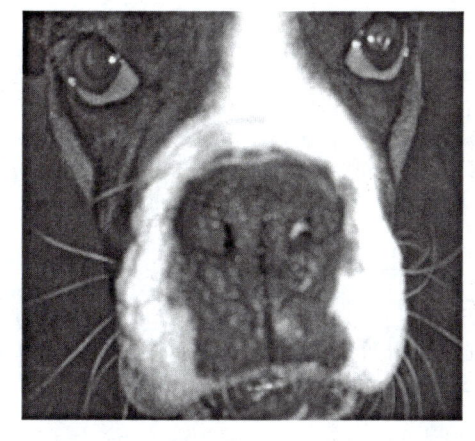

Systems and balancing and reorienting are well beneath the limited scopes of anyone's awareness. Practitioners and dogs have no idea how, what, why, on what level, or even whether, their bodies are responding.

Whatever happens during a PetMassage affects the very foundations for their emotional and physical bodies. Even when we see no spontaneous changes in behavior, we know that some level of course correction has taken place. Shifts and changes will become obvious after your dog is given time to integrate his inner dialogue. The shifts your dog experiences engage him entirely and profoundly. Mind, body, and spirit, at all levels are more flexible and balanced.

Reactive movement massage

Whatever happens within the dog's body-mind is always a result of the intimate interaction between the dog and you, the one facilitating his PetMassage.

Think of PetMassage as a reactive movement exercise. It's a dance. For thirty minutes, you and your dog's focus are responsive and reactive to each other. It's a relationship. As with any healthy relationship, an important aspect of it is making the effort to being non-judgmental.

Non-judgment is often a difficult concept to put into action. When we observe a condition, in order to make sense of it, we compartmentalize it. We put in a context we can understand by defining it to ourselves. As soon as we have named it, labeled it, we have judged it. It's good; it's bad. He's healthy; he's diseased. He's clean; he's dirty. He's friendly; he's scary. These are all judgments.

Those of us who are nurses know how easy it is to fall into the trap of referring to patients by their condition. Our patient is not the broken hip in 205. She is a woman who has a name, a family, and a fascinating life story. She is in room 205 and is frightened because her hip broke. Labeling can humanize or dehumanize. The words we use influence how we will interact with our clients. Our definitions frame our intentions and determine our actions.

It is easy to fall into the cycle of defining a dog by his condition. "Hobbs is the dysplastic dog." "Molly is the seizure dog."

The symptom is not the dog; it is only the behavior. It is the dog's temporary *condition* which is out of balance. See your dog as 95 percent healthy with the symptom as an aberration.

If a dog presents as injured, in pain, paralyzed, obese, or lethargic, you will certainly feel compassion. That's natural. If you didn't care and weren't empathetic, you wouldn't be learning the skills of PetMassage.

Your dog presents his current scenario of his body-mind experience. You respond with your entire body-mind as well. Your session will take place in this particular shared moment of each of your lives.

In addition to learning to closely observe your dog's reactions, you will need to develop self-awareness skills. Your entire body becomes an instrument for therapeutic interpretation. Each of your intuitive, reflexive responses is the natural and correct complement to your dog's spontaneous request. Incorporating self awareness, your presence addresses the entire gamut of canine physical and emotional situations.

There is a wonderful phrase that a colleague used that made me feel so good about myself I was giddy. She said, "You are doing it exactly right."

We've learned from quantum mechanic hypotheses that the act of observing magnifies an experience. What one focuses on, expands. Paying attention to all your dog's reactions and responses will influence him from the way he cocks his head to his genetic memory.

A PetMassage is an evolving relationship. Nobody knows all the rules for perfect relationships. You bring your stuff to the table and your dog brings his.

Once you have entered into your dog's world, apply your skills and enjoy the moment to moment intimacy and revelations of the PetMassage experience.

Positional release

PetMassage positional release increases your dog's body's natural restorative abilities, by accessing his intuitive body wisdom. Positional release incorporates many of the skills you've already learned. It employs light to moderate traction, observation, and the technique of follow-on, which includes another skill, a form of self awareness called empathetic participation. PetMassage positional release offers a wide range of benefits including the noticeable decrease in muscle tension, increased range of motion and (as humans describe it) a reduction in pain in the soft tissue. It also stimulates, supports, and witnesses the inner dialogue necessary for emotional course corrections.

Positional Release shows the body how to comprehend its current patterns and initiate its course corrections. It is the deliberate placement of the body into various "positions," from which it can "release" tightness and restrictions. The fascia that is freed up in the process, has been restricting muscle and joint movement, so this is also called "myofascial release." Improving circulation and nervous system transmission, its effect is powerfully therapeutic.

Positional Release always starts from stillness. Your hands cradle a structure of the body, such as a joint or area of fascia, and slightly transition it from its presented holding pattern to a position that feels mildly unfamiliar. The body takes control as it shifts internally, experimenting with different ways of positioning itself, forming a new perception of what its optimal comfort could be. Positional Release leads the body to realize it has functional alternatives.

There are three components:
1) Compression to expansion or unwinding, 2) stretching to recoil and retraction or winding, and 3) follow-on, resolution/observation

Positional release:
Compression to expansion demonstrated on an appendicular joint

The first part of positional release involves bringing the elements of the joint, or area on the body, together and observing how they reposition themselves.

The pressure is extremely light. Visualize the tissue between your hands, simply inhaling. Even this lightest of touch and compression stimulates the nerve endings within the fascia. The compression creates a slightly unfamiliar sensation. The body intuitively attempts to move back to its habitual position. The elements within the joint move. They slowly begin to shift, and rotate, and expand. The tissues realign themselves into a more comfortable position. This is called "moving to a place of comfort."

Body mechanics
Positional release compression to expansion
Place your Mother hand on the underside of a joint, such as the carpus, wrist, the active hand gently grasping the skin and coat, distal to joint, closer to you. Hold the limb in its natural position for several seconds; and then ever-so-slightly, reduce the space between the ends of the bones of the joint.

This is a subtle movement. The pressure is light, just enough to sense that the tissues are just a tiny bit closer to each other. The light touch compels the dogs to participate. The elements within the wrist, work to establish a sense of closure to light touch and completes the connection by expanding out to meet your hands. The lighter your touch, the more powerful your dog's release will be.

When you gently compress the gap, your dog's body learns something new about itself. As soon as the fascia realizes that it has been holding back it pleasures itself with a little sigh.

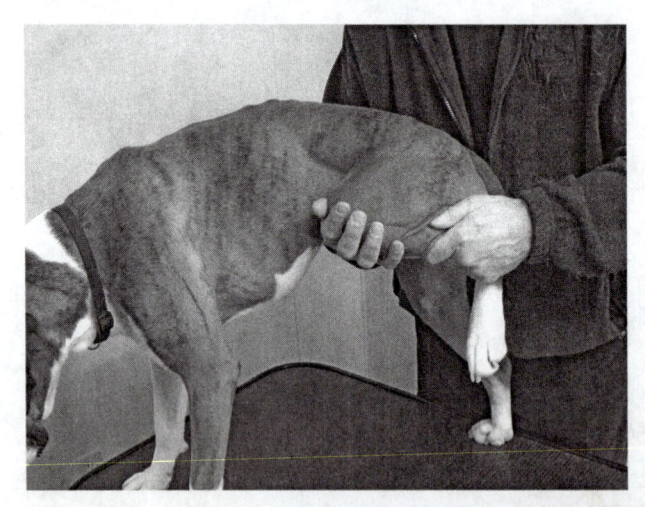

Note that in these illustrations, the movements are very small. You are developing a new sense; a new way of experienc-ing your world. It takes practice to be able to sense these movements.

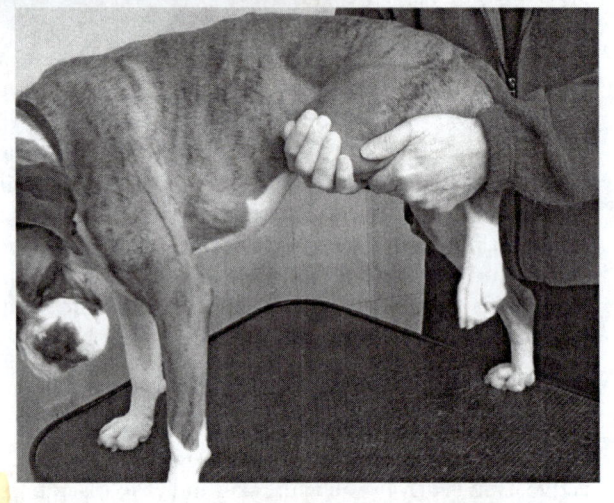

The sensation that you will feel in your active hand is a gentle push back, as if the body had been holding its breath and is finally able to exhale. The sensation that you will feel in your Mother hand is increased heaviness, as the body releases its need to control.

Repeat the compression to expansion three or four times. As you continue, you will notice that the movements come quicker. This is partly because the tissues are warmer, partly because they are feeling more freedom of movement, and partly because you are learning how to feel for this type of movement.

Unwinding is another term for this push back. Unwinding is a process in which the elements between your hands explore possibilities for movement. The first tentative push back is the body's effort to return to the position that it had been holding. The push backs that follow, assess and discover how it feels in alternative positions.

Unwinding is solidly based in anatomy, physiology and kinesiology. PetMassage exploratory unwinding is supported with observation and hands-on (mechanical) reinforcement.

The push back movements you feel may be the simple responses of the bones, ligaments and capsular tissues to your pressure. This is the simple version. In the larger picture, they are acting like tiny holograms, releasing restrictions held within the tissues of other parts of the body; in the extremities, in the pelvic girdle, along the spine, in the neck, and/or among the cranial bones.

This technique can be applied over any joint, any series of joints, and over areas of fascia that appear tight, restricted or out of balance.

Positional release compression to expansion triggers the dog's body to make its own choices. So, it is not only appropriate for overly tight limb joints. It is also effective on overly loose areas anywhere on the body.

Actually, any area that is not working in perfect accord with its adjacent tissues, can. with positional release, be stimulated and encouraged toward balance and more comfortable movement.

Positional release: Stretching to initiate recoil, demonstrated on the head, neck, trunk and pelvis

The second part of positional release slightly separates the elements of the joint, or area of fascia, and observes how they move back toward each other. This time you will experience "winding," a slightly different quality to the winding push back.

This time, the elements within the joint, or the parts of the body between your hands, seek and discover new places of comfort from a slightly expanded position.

Assume the same hand positions, with your Mother hand supporting and your active hand monitoring a joint, such as the stifle pictured here. This time, support the thigh and apply gentle traction to the lower leg, guiding it into about one-eighth inch of stretch. The elements within the joint capsule are being expanded into the slightly unfamiliar, more open position. The memories that are stimulated in the stretch will be different from those that would have been triggered when the movement facilitated closing. Closed memories would be restrictive, retractive, and pressure based. Open ones will be about expansion, opportunity, choice and empowerment.

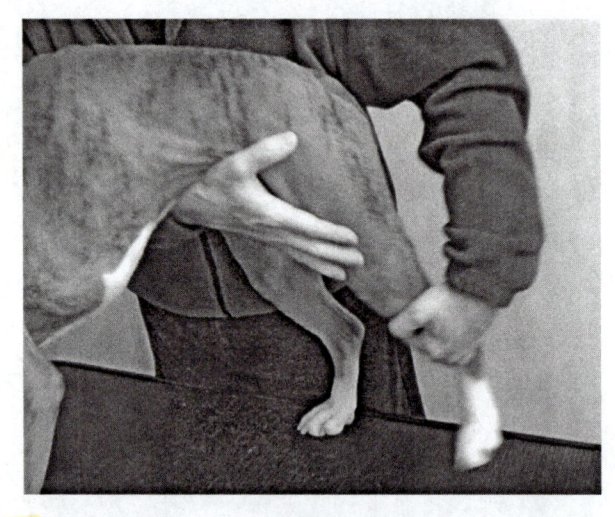

Support the body's pull-back intention, as it moves to retract to its normal pattern. Maintain your gentle grasp with your active hand, and when you feel the slightest inclination toward recoil, release the tension. Do not let go. Flow back with it, observing how it slides back over your Mother hand. Repeat three or four times. The angulations and power of the movements change with each return. This is winding, a type of exploration of movement. The body is exploring various patterns before it decides which one to choose.

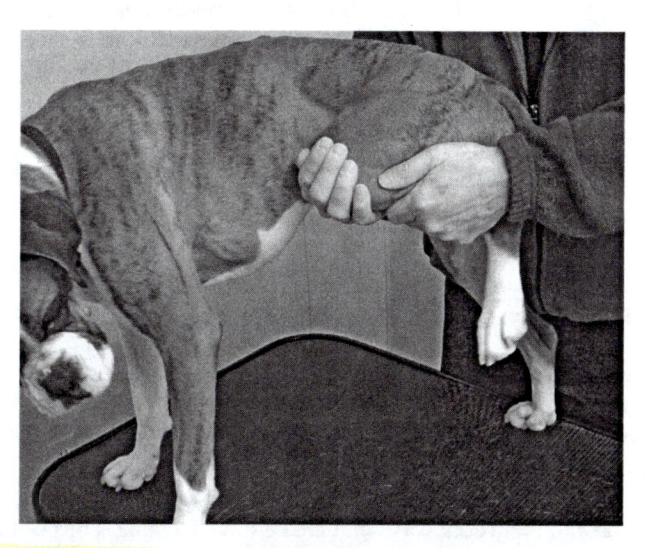

Stretching, or expanding, affects the nerve endings within the tissues. It elongates the space, shifting the pressure and the distribution of fluids within joint capsules. From this position, the elements within the joint contract, as the body intuitively moves back toward its normal holding pattern. Through the process of repeated expansion to recoil, the fascia slightly realigns. The new position is freer, more comfortable.

This new position feels like it has arrived home after a long time away. The sensation you feel in your active hand is gentle collection, as if the body has taken in a fresh tiny new breath, which it has. The motion that you feel may be as elegant as the way a rubber band feels when it is stretched and it returns back to its original size.

Apply this technique at the base of the tail (the entire spine, recoils and unwinds), over the hips, the stifles, hocks, toes, over the shoulders, on the ears, and across the back. Your new understanding of the way tissues move can be applied to all your vectoring, skin rolling, and joint mobilization. It will heighten your PetMassage experience.

You've witnessed, or rather, felt, how the body responds both in the compression to expansion and the stretching to recoil. Both of these techniques encourage the dog's body to notice how it is feeling, and if it discovers that there is a better, or more comfortable position, to choose the alternative.

All of the unwinding and winding that you've felt has been in the fascia. We've discussed the role of the body fascia, in all its solid, liquid and gas forms. Recall that it contains and coordinates all the organs, the muscles, fat, nerves, all the body systems, and the perceptions and memories of everything they've ever experienced. It is a vast network within which all of the systems of the body communicate and coordinate with each other. Your dog's toenail, at some level, knows how his pancreas is functioning, how his tail is moving, what his eyes are seeing and how secure he feels.

So, when you put traction on a toenail, you are stretching the eyeball.

There is more to the body than the physical. There is the ever-important and omni prescient emotional.

The dog's body retains its memories in the fascia as well. These are the memories of all its emotional references that are connected to its body positions and movement patterns. Happy, sad, fearful, etc. emotions are all embedded there, beneath your hands, within fascia that surrounds and binds muscles.

The dog's body and mind seek ways that create more balance. The positions they move through do not only bring about more comfort, they source happiness, sadness, and all the other emotions.

Putting it together: the follow-on

Compression to expansion and stretching to recoil, activate many body memories and references. Each return, exploratory winding or unwinding, discovers, uncovers, or recovers an alternative position.

You've observed and supported the body-breath as you've felt the fascia sigh and gasp, push back and pull. You may have noticed that the movement you feel within the joint tends to want to continue. It moves until it rediscovers its own version of homeostasis.

The Follow-on is the continuation of what you have observed. It adds amplification and flow to the earlier two individual movements. You will begin with the processes you've just learned and support the body's intuitive resolution of its exploration of movement.

Follow-on continues the compression to expansion initiative, *slightly exaggerating* the stretch. Then it continues the stretching, observing its recoil, *slightly exaggerating* the recoil. Your hands "follows on" the movements originating from the tissues. Now your dog can have slightly more generous opening and closing experiences.

One part of the position flows release into the other, releases and washes back. It is a gentle ebb and flow, ebb and flow.

Just as a straight line is an anomaly in nature, your Follow-on movements gently twist, curl, coil, or slightly rotate. There will also be tiny curves and figure eights. They seldom move directly in or out.

Notice the descriptive terms here: *gently, tiny, ebb,* and *flow.* These are very subtle movements that you will only be able to sense if you know what to feel for; and that comes with practice.

After three or four cycles moving in and out, they eventually come to rest and stop. When this happens, pause, maintaining your light supportive grasp and take two or three comfortable breaths. Your breathing sets the realignment. It is as important as the release.

How long does each area of the body take to realize its resolution? Each situation, like each dog, and each collection of your dog's emotional baggage, is unique. So, each will have different needs and will elicit different internal connections. Some will take as little as fifteen seconds; some, several minutes.

If you are not sensing movement, it does not mean it is not there. It is always there. It just means that you, meaning your body or mind, is getting in the way and blocking your open reception.

So what do you do? Focus on your breathing until your inhalation and exhalations are regular and your pulse is calm. Shift your weight, moving your center of gravity from one leg to the other. Often, shifting your weight modifies the unconscious body language signals that may be hindering your communication with your dog.

Continue to practice and observing will become easier. Functioning at this level is a learned skill, using muscles that you have not yet developed. With repetition, you will learn to become more observant and intuitive. You will develop muscle memory.

The follow-on is the most interactive part in the PetMassage process. Follow the movements as they continue in the dog's body, whatever they are and wherever they go.

Feeling the love: shifts, internalizing releases

PetMassage Positional release gently urges the dog's body to seek and discover its inner balance. How do you know when something happens?

We've seen how your observation plays an important part in the process. Monitor the dog's body as it moves from its contracted or expanded positions. Sense its confusion. Sense its power and empowerment. Notice how it settles into its new place of comfort. He may yawn, or shake; lick his nose or stretch, jerk his body or twitch. He will do everything he can to adjust to his new body education. You are now tapping into the dog's reservoir of body wisdom. Whatever movements that are internally initiated, you validate with your observation.

You felt it and know it, right along with the dog.

There is another element that you can do that will support the movements you sense even more profoundly. You can experienced it.

The sensations that you have of your body are your only real gauges to know that your dog is processing when his signals are too subtle for your conscious radar. Pay attention to the teensy tiny physical and emotional shifts that occur within your body.

Empathetic self-awareness is your guide. It is your proof that something is shifting. You are already supporting your dog's healing process with the pheromones that you release. Now, you can magnify their effect by noticing your physical and emotional variations and shifts.

This is a little exercise in multitasking. While you are following on the dog's body-breath and fascia, direct your observations inward. While you observe how your dog is responding to your various techniques, notice how do you feel in your body? Do you feel anxious, or confident? Do you feel breathless, sneezy, happy, bashful, dopey, grumpy, or docked?

Exaggerate your internal visualization of whatever movements that you feel. You may sense your body's empathetic physical winding or unwinding.

- You could feel motion in your chest or stomach or in the floor beneath your feet.
- You could feel a surge of power or weakness in your heart, your legs, your arms, or your fingers.
- You could feel winding, tightening or unwinding, unraveling in your shoulders, your stomach, your intestines, your colon, your pelvic floor.
- You could feel twisting or unwinding slowing down or speeding up anywhere in your body.

Allow your body to move into the patterns you feel. Keep your hands on your dog and dance with your feelings.

You may feel
- vertigo
- light headedness
- spontaneous bloat or gassiness,
- headachy
- fatigue
- increased energy
- your mind wandering

Hopefully you will not be having the same effects as your dog. Your issues are different; not sore hips, overt barking, separation anxiety, or housebreaking. However, the fact that you are processing something, anything, is close enough. As you follow on the movements of your dog's body, observing them as they shift about, you both support each other's movements toward your individual versions of balance, awareness and comfort.

Witnessing by itself is powerful. It is even better with its added value of sympathetic processing. This gives both of your inner puppies opportunities to make progressive choices. Your focus on self is the element that makes PetMassage so powerfully effective as a treatment.

Pay attention to your own thoughts and feelings. A cell phone ringing is enough to instantly disconnect you physically and emotionally. So, turn off your cell phone, your radio, your television, and anything else that might create a distraction. Restrict other dogs and people from your area while you are facilitating a session.

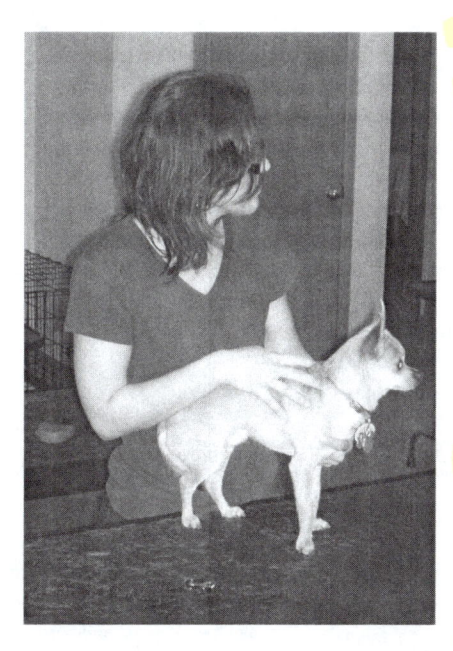

If you notice your mind is wandering, and it will, such as thinking about where you left your keys or what you need to purchase on the way home, maintain your physical connection with the dog with your hands, and focus your attention on the thought. Thinking about the thought separates you from it and diminishes its influence. Visualize a soap bubble around the thought and watch it float away. Let it go and refocus your breathing and attention.

Make sure it is your thought. We often recycle our thoughts. We repeat them or reconsider them in a different light. Our thoughts are our own unique patterns. We recognize them. We own them. They are who we are. We live in their framework.

The alpha state that you experience during positional release can open your mind so that it makes connections that had not been there before. It can make you more receptive to your natural creativity. In that case, pay attention to your thought and see how it has arisen from imaginings you've already had.

Sometimes, an image or feeling will surface which is not yours. You will know it by its strangeness; its lack of context. This is a new thought-experience. That is, your emotional or physical responses to the image are confused. You could be tapping into another's inner conversation. In the context of this intimate connection, the thought or image could be the dog's.

During a workshop, as I held a Rottweiler's paw, I observed the image of a long gray wooden walkway leading out to a boat dock over still water. I don't own a boat and have no interest in floating around swatting mosquitoes, so it certainly couldn't have been my thought. I described what I saw to his person, adding that there were no boats tied up to it and that I felt a feeling of emptiness. His person shared that they had just sold their boat and that her Rottie used to enjoy going out in it with her. He missed his boat! That must have been what was on his mind; and what he was processing.

Students are amazed at what they can feel and how gentle their touch must be. One workshop student documented that doing positional release work has "changed her life".

Human clients are amazed by the profound and lasting changes that they feel. Positional release has lasting effects in many aspects of a dog's life, improving quality of movement, digestion, and sleep and play patterns. Dogs consistently show spontaneous releases and rebalancing.

At dog agility and flyball competitions weakness and soreness that hindered movements often appear to evaporate. With PetMassage positional release our canine athletes perform better, faster and safer.

These are just some of the effects of positional release

- Paw
  Increases trust, comfort, confidence
  Decreases apprehension, fear
- Joints
  Assists dog's body to explore and chose among alternatives to joint alignment and comfort levels
  Increases ROM and flexibility to limbs, head and neck, spine, toes, increases blood circulation back to heart, increases lymphatic flow through large joints
- Fascia
  Creates an ambient environment for movement and healing
  Helps release holding patterns, habitual ways that a dog holds or carries his body, helps dogs release emotional holding patterns
  Gives dog permission to evoke deep seated course corrections
  Enhances dog's inner awareness
  Enhances connectivity within his body
- Skin
  Increases circulation, increases dog's awareness of his surroundings, increases sense of safety
- Coat
  Coat is first line of physical defense
  Increased blood supply supports the nerves attached to hair follicles in the superficial layers of the skin

> Take the time to feel the
> expansion or contraction
> response.

> Take the time to feel expansion or
> contraction
> of your heart.

> Take the time to feel expansion or
> contraction
> of your thoughts.

Stretching

One of the ways that we refresh our bodies is to stretch. It feels so good. All of the muscles are extended at once: the flexors, extensors and synergistic muscles. Of course, stretching is a natural movement for dogs. It's obvious they enjoy stretching as much as we do.

PetMassage stretching is always as an extenuation of the movements of positional release. The stretch, or extension of the limb or trunk, is always internally directed; initiated from the dog. PetMassage assists the stretch as it begins. As it unwinds, supports its movement, slightly extending it as body breath.

Even this gentle --and minimal--PetMassage stretching is a strength and toning exercise for muscles. It has these benefits:

- Increased blood flow
  Helps to warm-up muscles, increasing their blood flow and improving circulation.
- Relaxation of the massaged muscles
  The muscles are more relaxed. This is particularly helpful when you are about to stretch those muscles. It can also help relieve painful muscle cramps.
- Removal of metabolic waste
  Improved circulation and blood flow helps to remove waste products, such as lactic acid, from the muscles. This is useful for relieving post-exercise soreness.

Stretching can be a large movement, such as an entire hind leg straightens and flexes. See the photographs on pp. 189-90. It can be so small it is unnoticeable, i.e., blinking, widening the tissues around the eyes, straightening a toe, or distention of the anal sphincter.

Stretching helps your dog by

- enhancing physical fitness
- enhancing ability to learn and perform skilled movements
- increasing mental and physical relaxation
- enhancing development of body awareness
- reducing risk of injury to joints, muscles, and tendons
- reducing muscular soreness
- reducing muscular tension
- increasing suppleness due to stimulation of the production of chemicals which lubricate connective tissues
  [Ref:www.cmcrossroads.com/bradapp/docs/rec/stretching/stretching_5.html #SEC44]

Yawn

Often, a full-body stretch is embellished with a yawn. The yawn reflex provides a "rush of oxygen" to the brain. The whole body participates to support this work for the respiratory system. The neck elongates, the jaw opens wide, the forelegs reach foreword, the spine arches, stretching and stimulating all the muscles, ligaments and fascia attached to it.

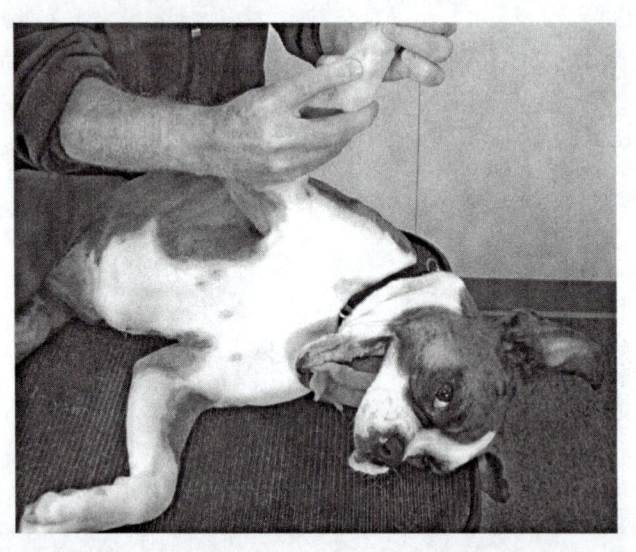

The yawn has psycho-social meanings, as well. Yawns, are contagious. One person (or dog) yawns and others follow. It invokes the feelings of relaxation, calm and refreshment. They are some of the most important signals we send to each other. Yawns can be warning signals [Darwin]. They can signal confusion; yawning might be a herd instinct. The yawn serves to synchronize mood in gregarious animals, similar to the howling of the wolf pack

[Schürmann]. or they can have a calming effect to defuse a volatile situation [Rugaas].

Your dog will yawn often during his/her PetMassage. This is
- a signal that he is relaxing and is encouraging you to join him
- an uptake of breath locking a memory of a muscle pattern
- an increase of Oxygen to the blood to facilitate more releases; alters the Oxygen: CO_2 ratio in the area of the table.

Consistent, balanced breathing, reinforces your presence and intention. Your breathwork provides, not only a model for your dog to follow, it structures the PetMassage.

Holding your breath, the opposite of a yawn, restricts and stifles your circulation. It effectively disconnects you from your dog. Support all of your dog's stretches with your breath.

Fascia

Think of the body as a single fascia membrane that includes all the muscles, organs, ligaments, bones, nerves and fluids. Fascia is a type of connective tissue that surrounds every muscle, bone, nerve, blood vessel and organ of the body. It is the fascia of stem cells that is the differentiating factor. Fascia forms sheaths for groups of muscles to function together. The ends of the sheaths are the tendons that connect the contractile part of the muscle to bones.

The recent work of Tom Myers, [Anatomy Trains] has documented a network of myofascial slings that span the length and breadth of the body. There are twelve of these fascia tracts, or meridians. They connect the body dorsally and ventrally on several tracts, running medially and sagittally. They also spiral and wind so that the entire body operates as a whole. No part is totally independent of the rest of the body.

These slings "have direct implications for posture, compensation patterns, and how pain expressed in one part of the body can actually be caused by strain in another part." [Myers]

Excess wax in one ear affects the way a dog holds and moves his entire body. The tension and/or comfort in a toe, affects movement of the head, the spine, weight bearing of the hips and tail carriage. Flea itching, fly bites, allergies, digestive disorders are all irritations of the fascia and its contents that shift awareness from homeostasis to chaos.

Learn the terms and know enough skeletal and muscle anatomy to be able to visualize the shapes of the major fascia slings of muscle groups. You will be able to feel them.

Exercise: Moving with and without assistance of fascia
Hold your hand out in front of you with your palm turned toward the earth (prone position). Turn your hand over, leading the movement with your thumb, so that your hand is supine, facing upward. How comfortable was this movement?

Return your hand to the prone position. This time rotate your wrist leading with your little finger. Which of the two movements was easier, more natural?

Fascia

Fibrous mucous membrane covering, supporting, and separating muscles. It also unites the skin with underlying tissue. Fascia may be superficial, a nearly subcutaneous covering permitting free movement of the skin, or it may be deep, enveloping and binding muscles. [Taber's]

Fascia is the fibrous tissue between muscle bundles or forming the sheath around muscles or other structures that support nerves and blood vessels. Deep fascia refers to fibrous tissue sheaths, containing little or no fat, that penetrate deep into the body separating major muscle groups and anchoring them to the bones. Blood vessels, nerves, and the spinal cord are all covered by fascia. [Beck]

Twelve body systems within the fascia

All twelve of these systems of the body depend on each other and work together to maintain life, function, balance and healing.

PetMassage with an awareness of the locations and functions of each of the body systems. Your dog will sense your confidence and professional attitude. As your intentions become clearer, your dog's body becomes more receptive.

From a holistic perspective, each body system has a unique personality, a specific job to do, and a working relationship with the other systems. Body systems are so interconnected that massage of one system always influences all of the others. Paired off they become the familiar terms that denote synergistic functions such as neuromuscular, musculoskeletal, or myofascial.

PetMassage is applied with the intention of returning each system to its optimal position, and functionality.

Each system also has a physiological rhythm that can be in tune with and even matched with the rhythm of your touch and your breathing.

1. Integumentary system
   The skin covers the body like a glove. It is peppered with highly sensitive nerve endings that alert us to a broad array of tactile sensations. It is the largest organ of the nervous system. It is like a sensory cloak that dogs wear to protect them from sunlight, abrasions and noxious elements. Skin regulates temperature cooling the body through conduction and evaporation (sweating). Skin relies on tactile sensations for neurological development. Dogs' skin and coats help control heat loss and serve as protective barriers.

2. Lymphatic system
   Located directly under the skin lives a lacy network of superficial capillaries and nodes of the lymphatic system, a major player in immunity. It uses gravity and pressure caused by internal squeezing of tissues during movement. Every movement we make and every breath we take, pulls open lymphatic vessels, which alters their pressure, so they can pick up excess fluid and waste products. This mix is then pumped through a series of nodes where it is cleaned and ultimately drained back into the blood stream. Light rhythmic touch gently stretches and twists the skin to open superficial vessels. The *spleen* is the organ that produces and stores lymph. It is nestled up against the diaphragm and is affected by rate and depth of diaphragmatic movement (breathing).

   There are several bilateral major nodes:
   - Submandibular, under the mandible, jaw
   - Prescapular, in front of the shoulder blades
   - Axillary/axilla, armpits
   - Inguinal, groin
   - Popliteal, behind stifles
   - There are also nodes between the ribs, on both sides of the sternum, and in the joints on the ventral side of the vertebrae of the spine.

3. Muscular system
   Peel away the skin and we find a tight elastic web of more than 500 skeletal muscles wrapping the body. As the workhorses of movement, muscles lack a mind of their own; they merely carry out commands of the mind. In this sense, muscle patterns quickly become habitual.
   Most muscular activity is carried out subconsciously.

4. Skeletal system
   The skeletal system is one of the clearest and easiest to find of the body systems. Bones function as semi-rigid structural struts, attachment sites for soft tissues and fulcrums for motion. Without them, the body would resemble a worm-like blob, unable to stand and moving with amoeboid quality. Bones are rich in blood and nerves, they benefit from massage.

5. Circulatory system
   The heart pumps blood through thousands of circulatory vessels that permeate every nook and cranny of the body. Although massage is thought to improve circulation, it is impossible to manually push blood back to the heart. Massage can, however, increase local circulation in areas being massaged. PetMassage mimics and accesses several blood rhythms: repetitive compressions mimics the pulsing arterial

rhythm of blood; effleurage, long flowing strokes against the lay of the hair, has the affect of sweeping the venous blood back toward the heart, and static contact, stimulates the blood suspended in capillaries.

6. Respiratory system
Breathing to the body is as wind is to nature: it blows out toxins and brings in fresh air. Following the oscillating tide of the breath during PetMassage it can reorganize respiratory muscles, to gently mobilize the spine, open the ribs, and bring an underlying support to the shoulder girdle. The accessory breathing muscles are diaphragm, intercostals, upper traps and pectorals. The d*iaphragm is an important muscle. It's the primary breathing muscle and moves the lymph by massaging the spleen which is nestled up against it. Its bellows action changes the pressures above and below it moving the interstitial fluids* .

7. Nervous system
This is the master coordinator and regulator of all the body systems. PetMassage accesses the somatic nervous system, and the autonomic nervous system. It is a binary system with both functional and structural aspects The conglomeration of nerve cells living in the brain and spinal cord resemble bulbous jellyfish with a long tail. Long fibers grow off each cell body, bundle into cord-like nerves, branch from the spinal cord at each vertebral segment, and thread through bones, between ribs and within myofascia, on their way to the periphery of the body. The natural elasticity of nerves allows them to bend and stretch during movement. *Chronic pain often comes from habitual postural patterns that entrap nerves in tight tissues. The patterns can often be released by repositioning the bones that nerves pass across, stretching myofascia around them, then applying light neural traction to the limbs and spine,* aka PetMassage Positional Release. The hair follicles in the skin are each attached to erector pili muscles which are controlled by the autonomic nervous system. Nerves sensitive to touch, heat, movement, and moisture cause the individual hair muscles to contract or relax.

8. Digestive system
This is a highly specialized organ tube that begins at the mouth and ends at the anus, and fills the abdominopelvic cavity. Parts of the digestive system can have high tone (i.e., tight throat, clenched jaw or irritated bowel) or low tone (i.e., distended throat or abdominal viscera). Abdominal massages can loosen tight viscera, tone loose viscera, and drop distended viscera into the lower back. Organs are close packed in their cavities, wrapped in pockets of fascia suspended by ligaments. Torsion in fascial pockets can twist organs, causing indistinct discomfort and pain.

The Digestive system is highly affected by emotional stress and unfamiliar or poisonous bacteria.

9. Reproductive system
   Massage can help alleviate aches and pains in human pregnancy and inguinal work can unravel myofascial tensions associated with hernias and release groin pain caused by entanglements in male reproductive tubing. PetMassage for pregnant dogs is primarily for relaxation and comfort.

10. Urinary system
    Including the bladder, this round muscular sack lives above and posterior to the pelvic bone, responds well to massage that stretches fascia around it. The kidneys also respond well to touch. They are often stressed from overactive adrenals and tight lumbar muscles.

11. Endocrine system
    Endocrine glands regulate metabolism through hormonal secretions. They can be overactive or underactive, potentially leading to metabolic imbalances that require medical attention. The glands, which are associated with the chakras, respond well to energy work, vibration, scents, and sounds that either stimulate or sedate them, depending on their needs. The endocrine system affects deep yet powerful aspects of somatic experience. Research from psychoneuroimmunology reveals that positive thought, feeling and relationships boost immune function, whereas negative experiences have the opposite effect. With this knowledge, the physical and emotional environment we create for massage may have as much of a healing effect on dogs as does our touch.

12. Chi or Qi:
    The life force energy that maintains and coordinates all the systems. This is the connection we and dogs have with the eternal and with their internal self determination. Chi moves with the oxygen in the blood and with the air that we breathe.

PetMassage affects every system.

System	Techniques	Affects
Integumentary	All techniques	Circulation to coat, skin, nerves in superficial dermis, stimulates or sedates, comforts or irritates
Lymph	Light scratching, brushing toward the heart	Stimulating lymphatic drainage, reduce edema and pain associated with the pressure of inflammation-swelling
Muscular	Deep stroking	Enhances venous flow, helps relieve discomfort and tightness
Skeletal	Compression, joint mobilization, rocking, positional release	Increases blood flow to bones, increases flexibility in joints, strengthens tendon and ligament attachment sites
Circulatory	Superficial stroking and tapping, rocking, positional release	Increases movement of blood and its Oxygen to muscles, to brain. Supports venous flow and blood supply for organ function
Respiratory	Compression, deep kneading and joint movement cupping/percussion	Enhances airflow, breaks up the phlegm in the lungs, enhances range of muscle flexion and extension: chest, ribs, diaphragm
Nervous	All techniques can be used on head and/or along spine	Enhance flow of Cerebral Spinal Fluid (CSF), increases balance and sensitivity of somatic and autonomic systems
Digestive	Still-holding, stroking, scratching, rocking, positional release	Supports movement of food from mouth to anus. supports motility of gut and absorption in intestines
Reproductive	All techniques--Caution: do not manipulate the hocks during pregnancy	Supports the body's processing of nutrients, creates ambient internal environment for optimal health
Urinary	Still-holding, stroking, scratching, rocking, positional release	Supports the body's processing of nutrients, creates ambient internal environment for optimal health
Endocrine	All techniques	Supports the body's processing and distribution of hormones, creates ambient internal environment for optimal health
Chi	All techniques	Maintains life force: flows with the blood, with the Oxygen, with the spirit, with thought

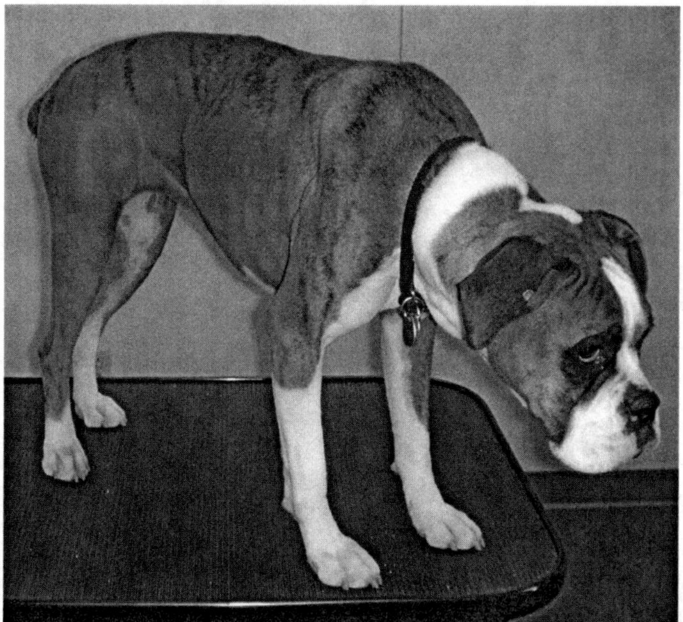

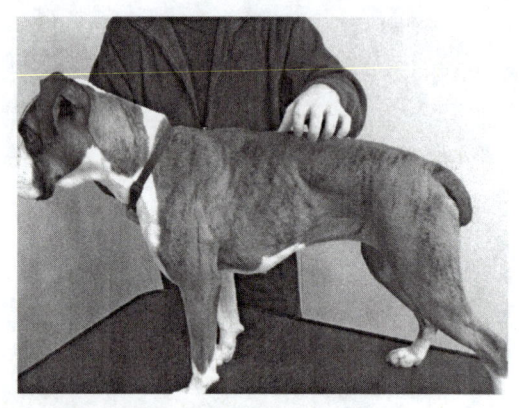

Connect the dots

Connecting the dots is the process of gathering your dog's awareness so that it is ready for your closing grounding ritual. Throughout his PetMassage, your dog has been observing your hands on his body wherever you have touched him. He is processing all the initial unwinding and exploration of movement that you have initiated.
Your dog can be in any position. He could be standing, sitting or lying on his side.

Body mechanics
Imagine a series of dots running on the dorsal and ventral midline of your dog's body. Lightly and quickly brush your fingers over these lines, moving from tail to nose, dorsally; and belly to nose, ventrally. This light brushing stroke brings your dog's attention back to midline.
From there it will be grounded.

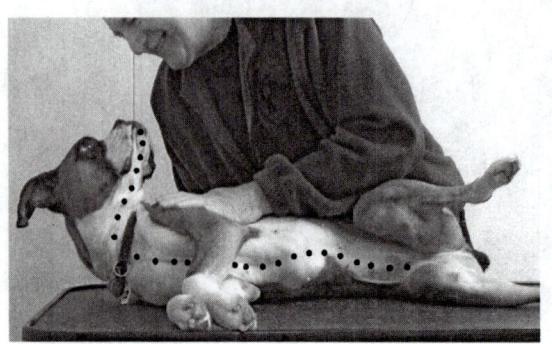

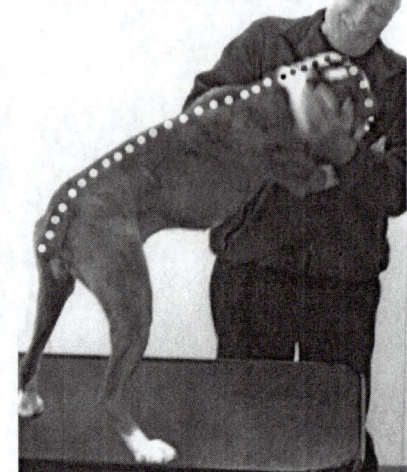

Grounding

All life springs from the earth and returns to the earth once it has run its cycle. The spirit, life force in your dog, is one with the earth. His life force is immortal.

While dog's bodies provide temporary accommodations, the life force continues, on its own frequency, to be aware. The spirit of the life force depends on the dog's limited lifetime of body-mind experiences to learn and evolve. Operating behind the scenes, it is part of the dog, and yet still connected with its source.

Your dog gets so distracted by all the things stimulating his active senses, he needs to be reconnected to the source of his power. That's where grounding helps. It is a physical reminder that he is a creature of Mother Earth. Mother understands. Mother loves us. Mother will take care of us. Mother will give us strength.

Grounding is the symbolic gesture that addresses the spiritual component of mind, body, spirit. Grounding gathers and channels the dog's life force back to it source, the earth.

The grounding movement collects the energy essences of the body that have just been stirred up during their exploration of movement and unwinding, and shows them that, on their soul level, they are safe and sound.

At the completion of the PetMassage session, lightly stroke the dog from nose to toes, sweeping your hands over the coat. Drag your palm down each leg and touch the ground (or the table) with it.

As you ground your dog, you are grounding yourself. Your respiration rate deepens and slows to a more comfortable and healthy rhythm.

Pheromones your body produces proclaim the calmness of your state of your consciousness. When your dog senses your breathing and smells the grounding chemicals in your skin and breath, he will feel more secure, knowing his leader is in a good emotional place.

Body mechanics
During grounding, your hands flow quickly over the body. You may use one hand as the active, while your Mother hand maintains your connection with the dog's body. Or you can use both hands at the same time. When using both hands, the grounding sequence is completed with two passes: one from the nose down both sides of the forelimbs, to the toes, and the second, from the nose, down both sides of the back and hind limbs to the toes. You do not have to ground the tail.

Breathing
Each grounding stroke is executed with an exhalation.

Inhale as your hands touch your dog's nose. Slowly exhale as your hands flow down over his body. While you are grounding your dog, between strokes, you may lift both hands off the body. A quick disconnect and reconnection with the second pass of grounding strokes prepares your dog for the final technique, the thymus thump and completion.

While it is uncertain that dogs understand, or care, about the concept of grounding, it has another benefit. This ritual movement gives you, the PetMassage provider, a sense of closure to the session. During the session, your inner puppy has been stimulated as well. It too could use a gentle reminder that it is safe and firmly rooted into Mother Earth.

A simple visualization will securely ground you and clear your energy. After you have completed the grounding ritual with the dog, pause. Breathe in and out two for several cycles while focusing on the bottoms of your feet and how they feel as the cushioned bridge between heaven (your body) and earth.

The post massage integration shake

The integration shake is a way to observe how the dog accepts and owns the PetMassage.

After your dog has completed his PetMassage session and is once again on the ground, notice how he moves. Observe him as he is standing, walking, turning and sitting. Dogs will often shake their entire bodies as if they are integrating all their reeducation experiences into their bodies.

Observe the shake to see if the dog shakes through his whole body. Notice if he only shakes to a certain point such as just the head, or just head and neck, or to mid back or entire body except for one of the rear limbs or tail.

The point where shaking stopped is a point of stasis. The flow has been interrupted and has not been able to travel past this point. This is an area you will want to revisit with additional PetMassage or encourage the flow in that area with skin rolling and positional release in the next session.

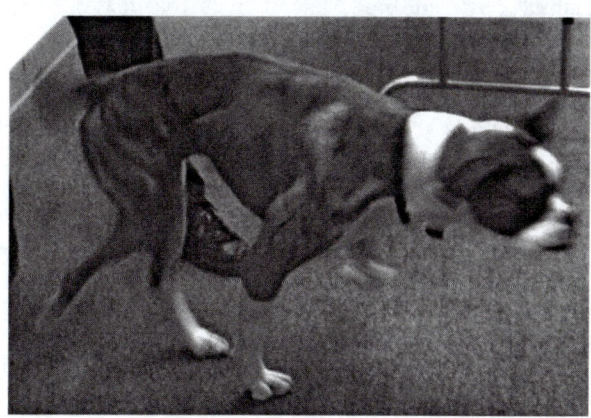

Body mechanics, part of body language

Keep your knees slightly bent, your back straight and vertical. Your head should be gently balanced on top of your neck. Remember not to slouch or roach your back leaning over your dog.

Be sure that you do not cross your arms in front of you. This is a signal that you are disconnecting, like a dog turning away. Any tension that you hold in your body restricts your blood circulation and is stagnating the flow of your Ch'i energy. When your energy flow is reduced your dog will respond, in kind. His energy level will reduce along with yours.

Be aware of what your dog may perceive as dominance movements.
Arm over withers, direct eye contact, excessive crowding, that is, not allowing the dog to have a visual line of escape; are all signals that dogs interpret as being aggressive. Your body posture and position tells the dog a lot about your intentions. If you approach the dog with your shoulders back, your back straight, and stand in front of the dog with shoulders square to her, you are projecting a dominant and domineering demeanor. Standing with your fists on your hips, the backs of your hands toward the dog is also a threatening gesture.

When you think about it, you'll see that this position, forces you into a square-on position. Your knees are locked, your jaw is thrust forward and the tension in fascia holding your neck muscles draws your mouth down into a scowl. Yes, I'd call that threatening.

If your dog's forelegs are rotated medially, the tops of the paws are more visible, the elbows are bowed out to the sides. This posture sinks the base of the neck into the chest and bulges the sides of the neck out, juts the chin forward and turns the dog's mouth into a menacing look.

Straight direct paths can be interpreted as menacing and confrontational. Curved paths project a softer, more feminine intention.

A more comfortable presentation is to approach from the side, or in a slightly curved path, and stand with one shoulder either dropped or pulled back, giving the dog the impression of a line of escape. Pulling the shoulder back is like a dog cocking his head to one side or sitting back on her haunches. It is a softer, gentler posture; one that is less likely to attack.

If you find yourself standing square-on to a dog, and we all do at one time or another, simply shift your weight from balanced on both feet to most of your weight on one side. This will effectively drop your shoulder to an acceptably comfortable level.

If you find yourself short of breath, open your posture so that your chest and belly are open and available. Straighten your back. Drop your shoulders into a comfortable position. Raise your chin and turn the corners of your mouth up into a gentle Buddha smile. Now you can breathe.

Where oh where

Where can you administer PetMassage? Probably a better question is where not? Let's talk about working on the floor, on a bed, and on a human massage table. I don't like any of these choices.

The floor is too low. It's also your dog's turf and although they feel the most at home on the floor it is there where they are also the most in control.

It took me several years to realize that it is not only awkward and uncomfortable for me to crawl around on the floor after dogs; it also restricted my ability to breathe. Whenever I am leaning forward, bending or twisting at the waist, my ribcage and my insulation press against my diaphragm, restricting my ability to fully inhale. Within a few minutes, I am out of breath. Without oxygen, my drug of choice, I tire quickly. I feel discomfort in my shoulders, back and knees, and cramping in my feet. I am hardly in a good physical or emotional place to provide support and love.

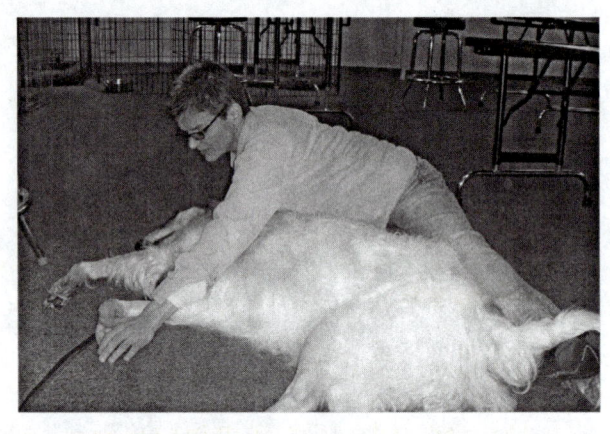

Giving your dog a PetMassage on a bed is also a very uncomfortable and unhealthy experience. If you were to stand next to the bed, your work surface would be too low and you will need to bend and stretch to reach your dog. We know what that does to you. Sitting next to the bed, facing it puts your body too far away and you will have to reach to touch your dog. Once again, you are compromising your breathing.

Sitting sideways next to the bed works if you only use one hand. In order to use both hands you will need to twist at the waist. Besides, most mattresses are so soft that your dog may stress his shoulders, elbows and wrists whenever he stands.

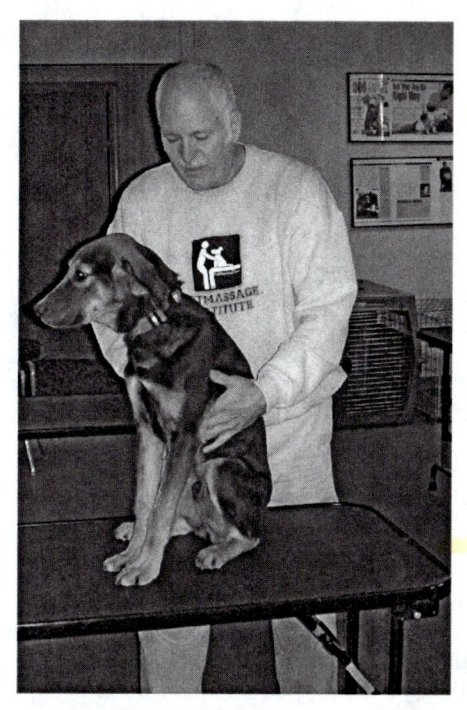

Working on a human massage table would give you the ability to move the dog above the floor, but not control the height. And to move around to reach the dog; it might be too awkward to walk all the way around a long table.

Human massage tables are great for dogs that are lying on their sides; but they are too soft for dogs that are standing. The cushioned surface causes strain and stress to their elbows and hips. If you insist on using your human massage table, firm the cushioning with a thick carpet or lay a board on top covered with a bathroom rug. Bath rugs work well. They have skid resistant rubber backings and are washable.

Your best workstation is on a sturdy dog grooming table. Your dog will be off the ground and at a level for you to work in comfort. The goal is for you to be able to comfortably access your dog's whole body without either of you having to stretch or strain your bodies.

A 2 x 4 foot table is the size work surface that we've found works best. It is a size you can easily move around and be able to reach his entire body. You can walk around the table. You can reposition his body so that it is comfortable to get to all the areas you want to access. You can keep your back straight and use correct footwork and body mechanics. It is also a convenient size to fold up and carry for PetMassage house calls.

Your PetMassage will be most effective when your dog feels safe. The table should feel stable and solid under your dog's feet. If you can stand on it and wiggle and still feel safe, then it will probably be safe for larger dogs. There are a lot of hundred and fifty pound dogs who need PetMassage. Most of the time your dogs will be in the standing position.

During his PetMassage, your dog will continuously move about. At various times during his session, he will be standing, sitting, lying on his side, on his stomach, and on his back.

Make sure he has enough room to readjust his body without falling off, for his safety; and, for yours. Plan for enough space around the table so that you can comfortably move around and rock and roll with his body.

Where you massage will depend on the size, disposition and personality of your dog. You may have to sit on the floor with your larger dog, or one who is afraid to get on the table. There are no hard and fast rules. Each situation will present differently.

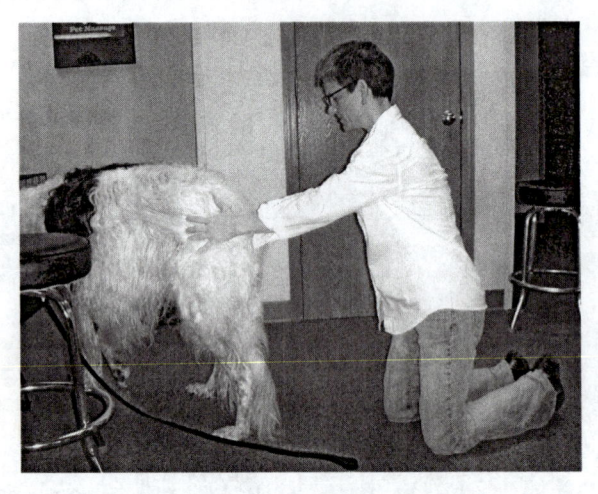

Whenever possible, for comfort and safety, PetMassage medium and small sized and all compliant dogs on your grooming table.

Wherever you choose to work be sure that your dog has secure footing. Avoid slippery areas such as tile, laminate or tightly grained, polished hard wood. These popular floor finishes are responsible for many dogs becoming lame and exacerbating hip dysplasia.

There are good reasons why many veterinarians choose to use slippery stainless steel examination tables. For them it is a good material. It cleans well, and the dogs that are put on it, have a hard time getting a secure grip with their paws. Uncomfortable medical examinations and procedures can be accomplished quickly while the dog is kept off balance. For our purposes, we want the dogs to enjoy their participating so carpeting on the table or floor, providing sure footing, is essential.

Now we know why carpets were invented: for PetMassage!

Safely assisting your dog onto and off the table

Practice moving your dogs on and off the table in ways that are safe, secure and comfortable. Good body mechanics are essential. When your dog is lifted correctly you send the message that you both are safe.

Always bring the dog as close as possible to your body. Hold him firmly, so that he feels secure and cannot wriggle away. Keep your back straight and lift with your legs.

If a dog is less than 35 pounds, 15 kilos, you ought to be able to safely pick him up and deliver him onto the table, without straining your arms, shoulders, and back.

When your dog is heavier arrange for him to mount the table from a raised platform or steps. Ideally, your dog will stand with his front paws on the table so that you can hoist his rear end up and he can walk forward.

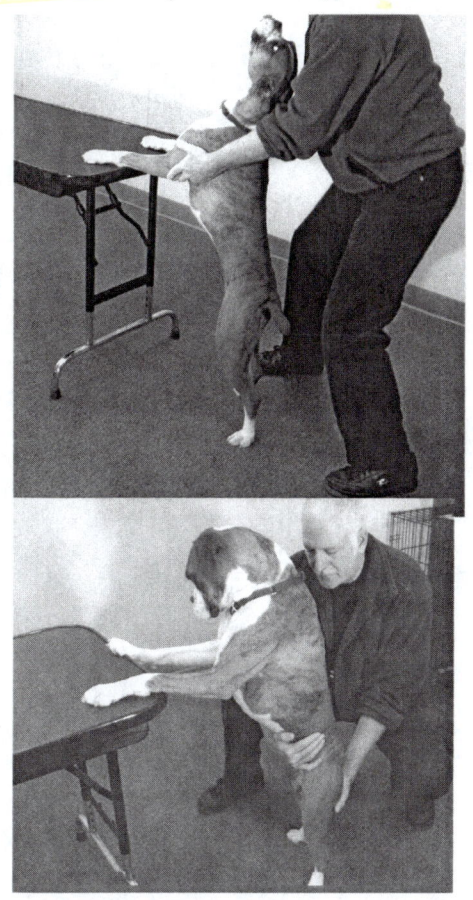

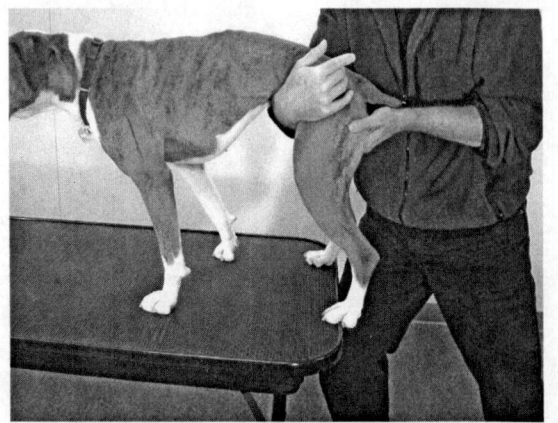

Assisting dog onto table

Assisting dog onto floor

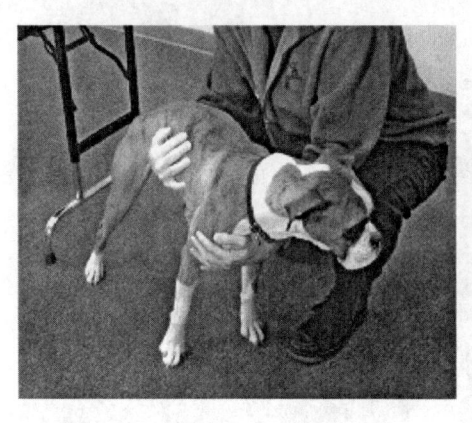

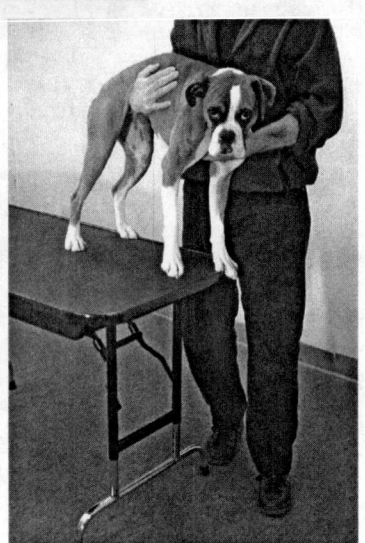

Table Manners	Table Manners
For your dog - No licking your face - No jumping up to put paws on your shoulders - No jumping off the table during a session	For you - Keep at least one hand on dog at all times - Pay attention - Keep breathing - Keep a smile on your face

Setting the scene: enhancements and distractions

It is not necessary to light candles and incense or use essential oil, aroma therapy with PetMassage. The only needs your dog has are for you to be present with him/her and feel safe and supported. Beyond that; minimize distractions. Turn off your cell phone, the TV, and restrict interested onlookers for the time you are having a session.

Restrict other pets who might wander into the area. This is your dog's special time and place with you. You'll both enjoy this privacy. De-pending on your dog's comfort and capacity for inward focus, you may, at your discretion, allow his/her guardian to observe; but not to touch their dog during the PetMassage.

Let's talk a little about the use of light and air and music in your PetMassage. Good lighting is important in that it creates an ambiance, a mood, and its characteristics can have a strong effect on your dog. Direct overhead lighting is never complimentary to our facial features. Your feelings about yourself are influenced by the light you are in. Again, your feelings will be transmitted through your hands. Your dog, who depends on the angles of the light to observe your body language is watching the lights and shadows of the contours of your face.

A smile in soft angled light may appear as a scowl with harsh overhead lighting. Florescent lights, especially the older ones, have a pulsing flickering quality. This "feature" has been shown to provoke seizures in people and animals with epilepsy. Incidentally, the red laser pointers that are such fun toys for cats to catch can also induce seizures.

The optimal lighting is sunlight, filtered through shades. The next best options are lamps with full spectrum lighting.

Air flow is important for your dog and for you. Stagnant air creates stagnation and sluggishness in both your bodies. If your objective is to increase circulation and flexibility, your work will be more difficult in a "stuck" environment. You must be able to breathe easily. Your dog must be able to breathe easily.

Your PetMassage relationship needs space to expand and contract, inhale and exhale, open, close and develop.

Dogs have a natural awareness of the movement of environmental energy in their environment. They could be Feng Shui masters.

If, during a PetMassage session, your dog shifts his position on the table, standing up, lying down, sitting, leaning, or turning to face into a different direction, he is simply aligning his body with a new current of energy flow. His environment is readily affected by sounds, vibrations, air conditioning and heater blowers, distractions from people, animals and motor vehicles, patterns and lights from windows, and food and especially, environmental aromas.

Dogs can even smell your thoughts. Consider that every thought you have evokes some level of emotional response. Happiness, sadness, peacefulness, confusion, certainty, anger, fear, confidence, frustration, satisfaction, love and hate. Your body reacts to each emotion as a means of protecting you from your daily saber tooth tigers, as part of your flight or fight response. The flight or fight response causes a surge of adrenaline and other stress hormones to pump through your body. This surge is the force responsible for mothers lifting cars off their trapped children and for firefighters heroically running into blazing houses to save endangered victims. [Bodysoulconnection]

Each of these hormones has its own distinct frequency and aroma. For example, the uric acid in the perspiration of a person in a calm and healthy state will have a different consistency and fragrance than if she had the flu, or was afraid, or infatuated. Dogs, with the sensitivity to detect aromas hundreds of thousands of times more than humans, can most certainly notice the shifts in the qualities of your perspiration as you are thinking. So, a simple daydream can shift the energy flow in the room.

Use aroma therapy as sparingly as possible. And then, only if you are absolutely sure it will enhance your PetMassage. A dog's sense of smell is much more sensitive than ours. Like any therapeutic tool, too much, will destabilize an environment, making it feel unsafe and uncomfortable. A little essential oil goes a long, long way.

Your dog needs to be able to smell you. Your presence and the aromas of your intention are what will enhance the time you share, not perfumes, diffusers and scented candles. Do not add anything that might get in the way of experiencing each other.

Aromas from bottles will distract from ordinary smells.

Another challenge for the use of aroma therapy is that we have no way of knowing what the appropriate dosage is, especially for dogs. We can extrapolate from our human experiences, but who can be sure how it will effect your dog? Even within a small group of humans there is a wide range of divergent responses. Dogs, cats, rabbits and horses all have different responses to similar aromatic frequencies.

Not all dogs react to fragrances, or anything else, the same. They are all individuals. Remember that essential oils have different effects on different individuals. Lavender, in essential oil form, applied directly to the skin, can be relaxing. It can also be poisonous or even carcinogenic. Echinacea, can stimulate the body's non-specific immune system and ward off infections. It can also trigger allergic reactions.

No agent and no one technique has universal applications. If you subscribe to the principles of "always promote safety," or "first, do no harm," then focus your attention and abilities on something you can measure, and you can know is working. That would be no-frill, hands-on PetMassage.

If playing music calms and helps you to center yourself, then play music. As far as I can know, dogs do not have specific tastes in music, although they do respond to the spirit of the sound. If the music is fast, loud, and exciting, it will excite you and your energy will transfer to your dog. If it is slow and dreamy, it will encourage you and your dog toward meditation.

If you play classical music that has a complex theme and development such as a piece by Bach or Mendelssohn, know ahead of time that you will be carried along with the emotional dramas the music evokes.

Whatever your experience is will be telegraphed through your hands.

The only precaution that I can suggest is to avoid recordings with nature sounds. Yes, it is true that our dogs are natural beings and love the outdoors; they also are distracted by the sounds of birds and crickets. Thunder storm cracks, crashes and noisy water dripping won't help your focus either.

In your practice, unless there is some noise that you want to block out, such as traffic outside the window, voices in the next room, or voices in your head, play no music. Concentrate on being present to listen to your new thoughts and the natural sounds coming from your bodies. You may not be able to catch the gentle *borborygmus*, tummy gurgle sound, over your cranked up old Dylan LP's. The gurgle is a sign of tension releasing in the body.

Establish PetMassage time for your own dogs to be at a time that is convenient to you. Dogs love their PetMassages and once they sense that there is a routine, they will hold you to it. One of my students complained that she is often late getting out the house in the morning, because she started PetMassaging her dog while she was getting ready for work. Her dog won't allow her out of the bathroom until he gets his PetMassage!

Before each session, ground and center yourself. Feng Shui (arrange your internal furniture for optimal energy flow) within and without. Your presence of mind creates a safe and secure, happy and healthy environment.

Choose or design an environment where you are most comfortable and can best have a sense that you are in control of your environment. This means reducing clutter and reminders of unfinished projects, like bills to be paid, messages to be returned, and records for your next client.

To sum up, ask and receive your dogs permission. Make sure that you are in a well lit, non-fragrant, breathable environment. Provide the PetMassage on a sturdy, secure table or raised, carpeted platform. Keep breathing and continue to have good body mechanics. These will ensure that you and your dog share the most positive PetMassage experience possible.

Sometimes, when you ask permission, the dog resists, indicating that he is not happy. It is possible that he's just not in the mood; but not likely. If he is asked correctly, with the right body language, he may be more willing to participate. The first and most likely scenario is that the resistance is coming from you. If so, regroup.

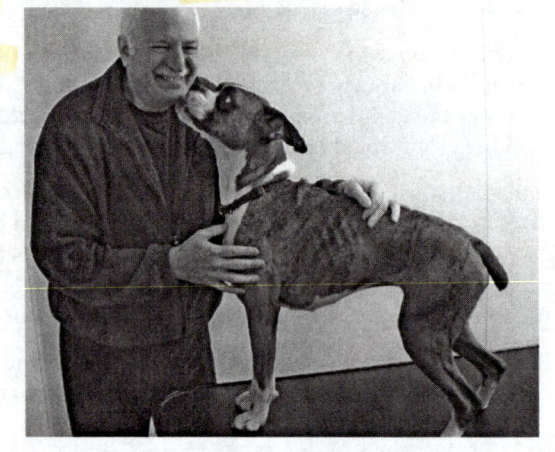

Quiet yourself.

Reestablish in your mind that you are safe and secure. When you change your perspective, everything around you, which is based on your thought-form, shifts. There is no reason to reconnect with your dog until you've regained composure.

The dog in your hands is more aware of your energy than you are. Observing your thoughts will significantly adjust the energetic body armor that surrounds you, your aura. Objectifying the thoughts and emotions that are running like a looped recording in your head will take most of their power away. As you become more available for your dog, your dog will be more receptive. He is acknowledging you as his leader and will synchronize his mood with yours.

Observe your breathing. When you've rediscovered your balance, feeling safe and confident, reconnect.

If you've determined the resistance is not coming from you, it is coming from your dog. He may be frightened, acting out, or yielding to his old emotional hooks and behavior patterns.

Spinning, growling, backing up and cowering are all recognizable signs you'll know when you see them. There is a natural desire to join up with the energy of the resistance to your overtures, to meet the energy you feel with a similar energy. Strength begets a strong response. Gentleness is met with softness. Anxiety provokes fear.

Your perception of your dog's resistance, and your dog's interpretation of your perception, could easily escalate an already stressed situation.

Make sure he knows you feel safe in his presence. Your quiet controlled presence may be an oasis of calm in your dog's chaotic world.

Putting it all together: Basic full body PetMassage

A PetMassage session

The elements and order for a PetMassage session
- observation of gait, comportment
- situating dog on table (body mechanics)
- permission
- breathing, connecting and releasing expectations
- vectoring over six channels
- assessment strokes over the six pathways covering the whole body
- Light: "Hi. How are you?"
- Medium: "Here I am to work with you."
- Deep: (stripping) "Here you are."
- head and neck: frictioning, skin rolling, tapping, thumb compression, rocking, joint mobilization, positional release
- on trunk and ribs: skin rolling, cross skin roll, scratching, clasp hands, cupping, rocking and spinal tapping
- legs and paws: frictioning, joint mobilization, scratching, positional release to stretches
- tail: compression, positional release, rocking
- re-assessment over the six pathways covering the whole body
- repeat vectoring over six channels
- connect the dots
- grounding
- breathing, disconnecting and thanking
- thymus thump
- assist dog onto floor (body mechanics)
- observation of gait and attitude
- integration shake
- elimination, hydration
- thoughts, imaging, documenting

The following is a demonstration of the full session. Your dog will decide how long the session will last, what he wants to focus on, and when he has had enough. Your PetMassage may or may not include everything listed.

Be aware and open to your dogs and their needs.

During assessment and all palpation, if you discover anything out of balance, assist the dog in reestablishing his balance, his intention toward wellness. Focus on the positive. Visualize your dog in a state of absolute happiness and comfort. Sense and re-enforce what works, <u>not</u> what's not working.

How are you defining your dog. Is he 96% perfectly healthy but has a dysplastic hip condition, or do you refer to him as the "dysplastic dog." The words you use shape the images you send. Your descriptions are affirmations. They define the dog to the dog. We know that dogs will do whatever they can to please us and validate us. So, dogs will strive to become your affirmative statement/vision.

Good body mechanics will maintain your connection and connectiveness with your dog.

- Breathe.
- Whenever you feel strained, stressed or out of breath, correct your posture.
- Keep your hands in front of your shoulders.
- Hold your elbows close to your sides.
- Have your thumbs directed upwards.
- Do not cross your arms in front of your body.
- Do not stand square-on to the dog. Angle your body or drop your shoulder.
- Each independent action is important and facilitates its own response. And no action goes unnoticed! Your unconscious, "busy" fingers that pet and scratch without purpose, only distract.
- Maintain contact with your mother hand throughout the PetMassage (both hands function as both active and mother).
- Pay attention to the connection that your feet have with the ground beneath them.
- All movements, even the tiny ones, begin and end with your footwork.
- Pay attention to how your dog is moving on the table.
- Pay attention to the signals your body is sharing with you.

Observation

Notice how your dog moves. How comfortable is he while sitting, standing, lying. Notice any unusual behaviors such as cowering, double tracking, sway back, and limping. Notice the sheen and quality of the coat.

Walk with the dog for a few minutes, getting a sense of his gait, rhythm, personality and to establish a rapport.

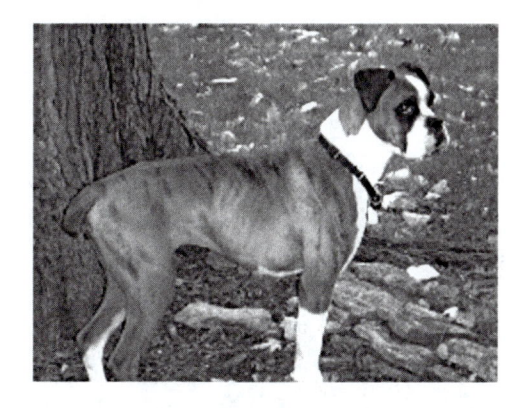

Situating dog on table

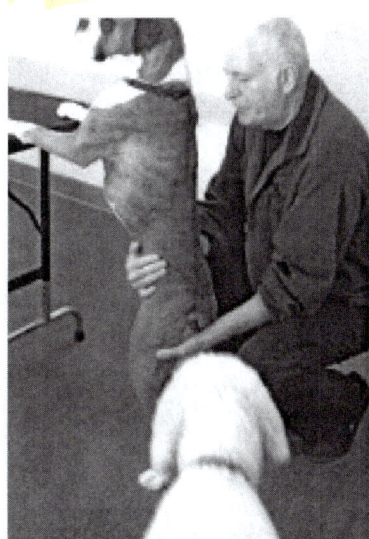

Keeping your back as straight as possible, bend your knees and collect the dog. Keep his weight as close to you as possible and lift with your legs. Walk him onto the table.

Permission

Ask you dog for permission to PetMassage. Observe his body language for your answer.

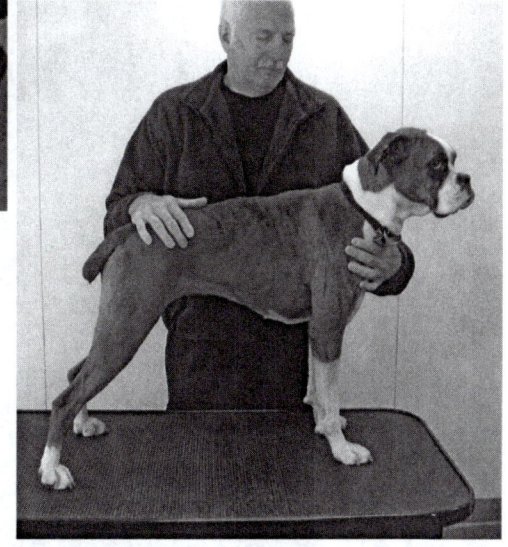

*Breathe,
connect and
release expectations.*

Vectoring

Take your time, use still-holding with observation. Breathe easily and rhythmically. This sets the mood and intention for the session.

Chest and mid back

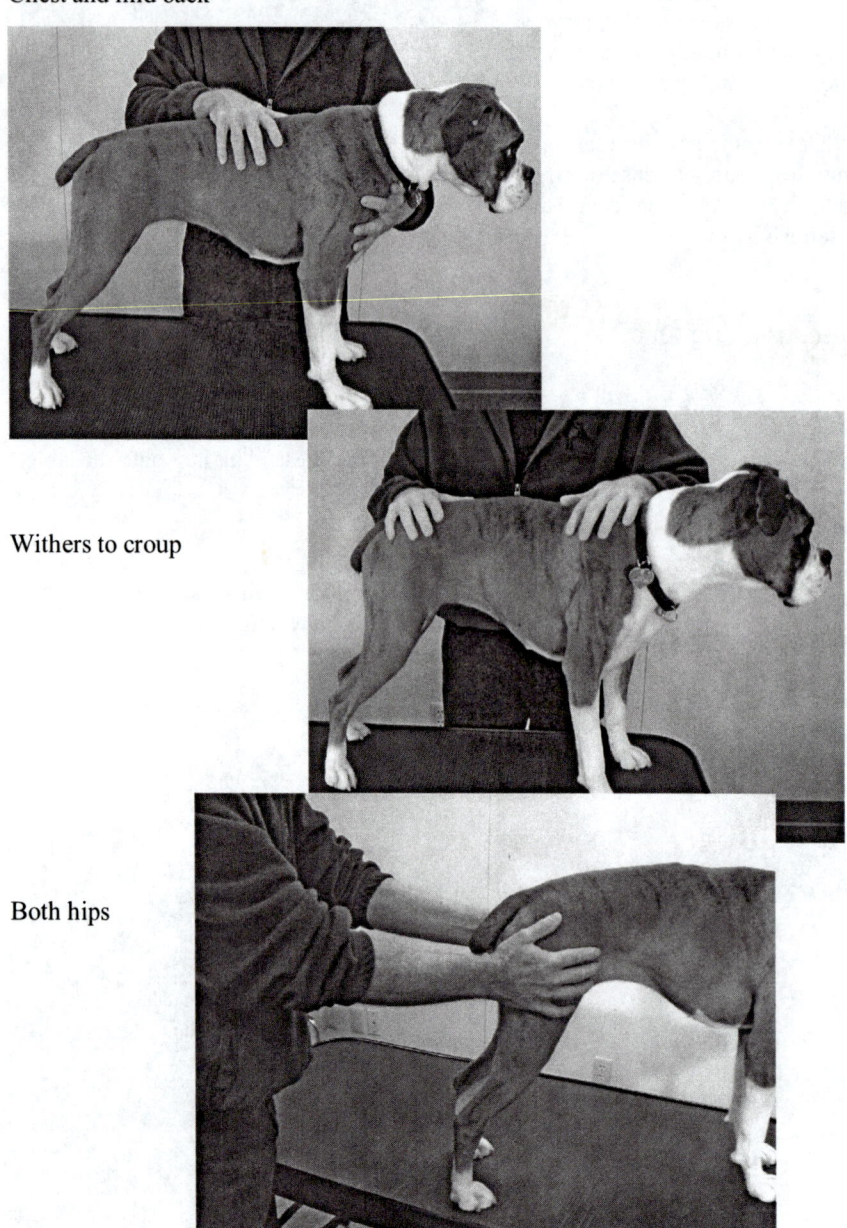

Withers to croup

Both hips

Sides of ribs behind the elbows (Heart to heart)

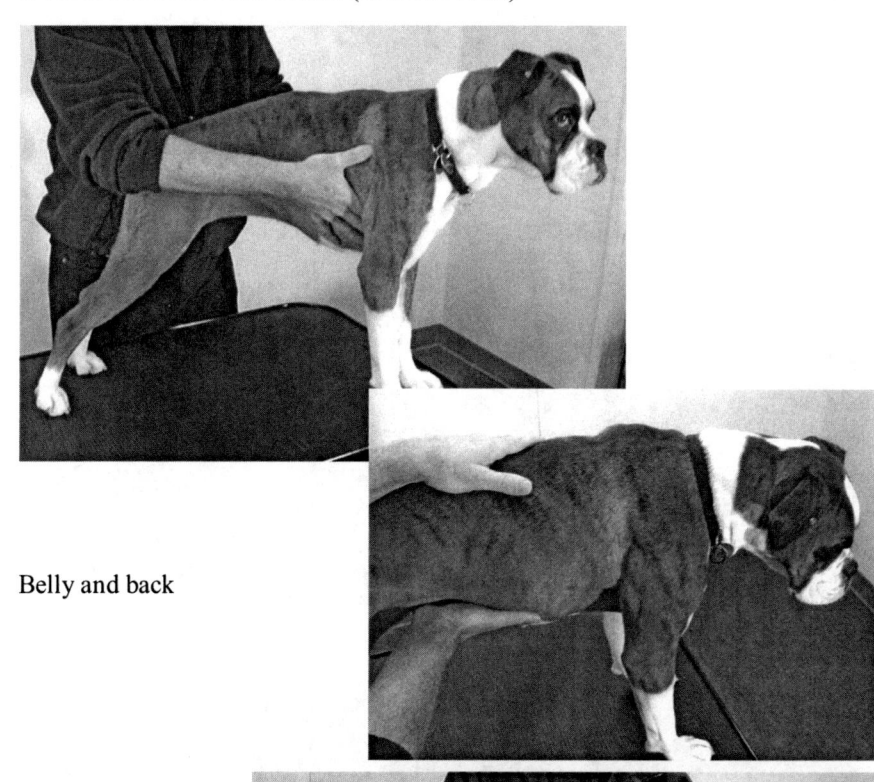

Belly and back

Mid back and chest

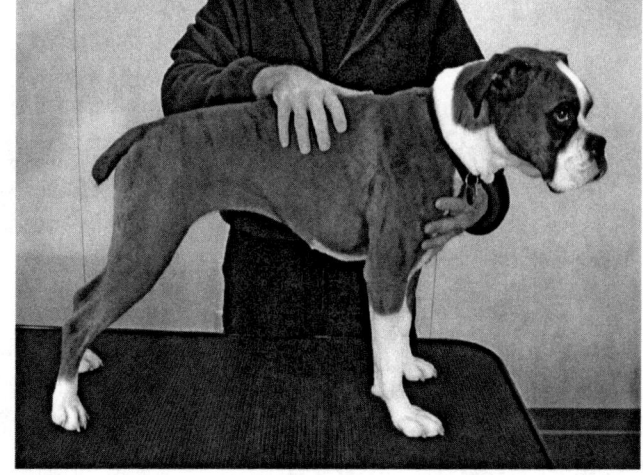

ART AND ESSENCE OF CANINE MASSAGE
PETMASSAGE™ FOR DOGS

Assessment strokes
flow over the six pathways covering the whole body. Observe how your dog respond to your touch at each level.

Three strokes: Light: "Hi. How are you?"
　　　　　　　　Medium: "Here I am to work with you."
　　　　　　　　Deep: (firm) "Here you are."

Dorsal line nose to tip of tail

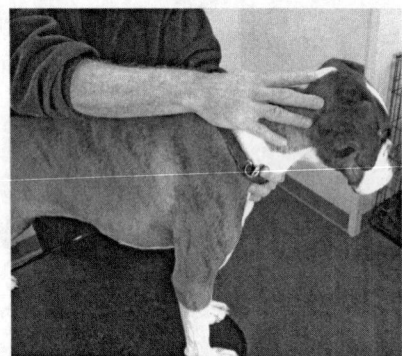

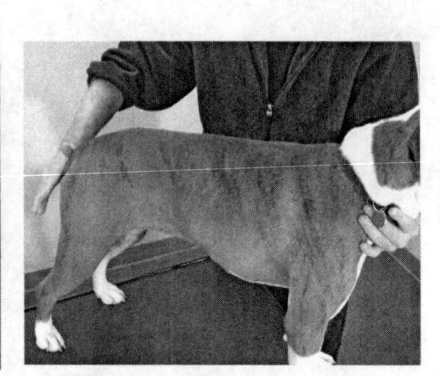

Head and right foreleg, nose to toes

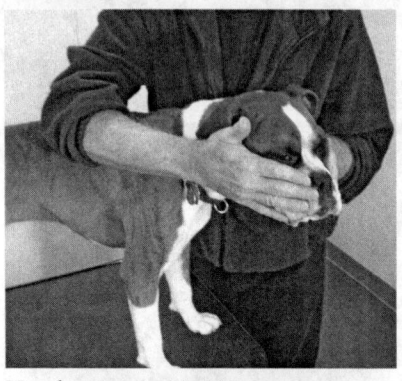

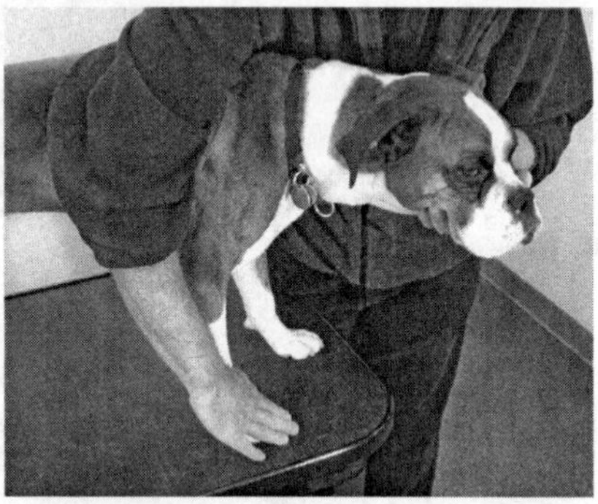

Head and right hind leg, nose to toes

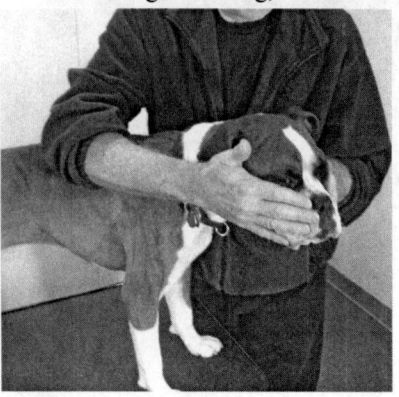

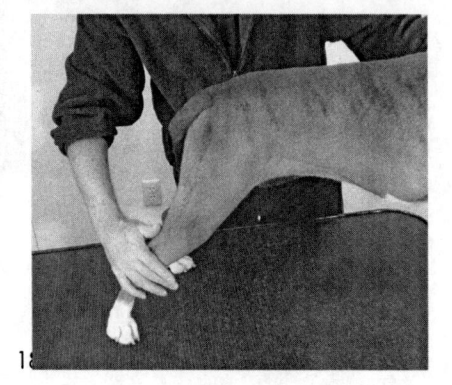

Head and left foreleg, nose to toes

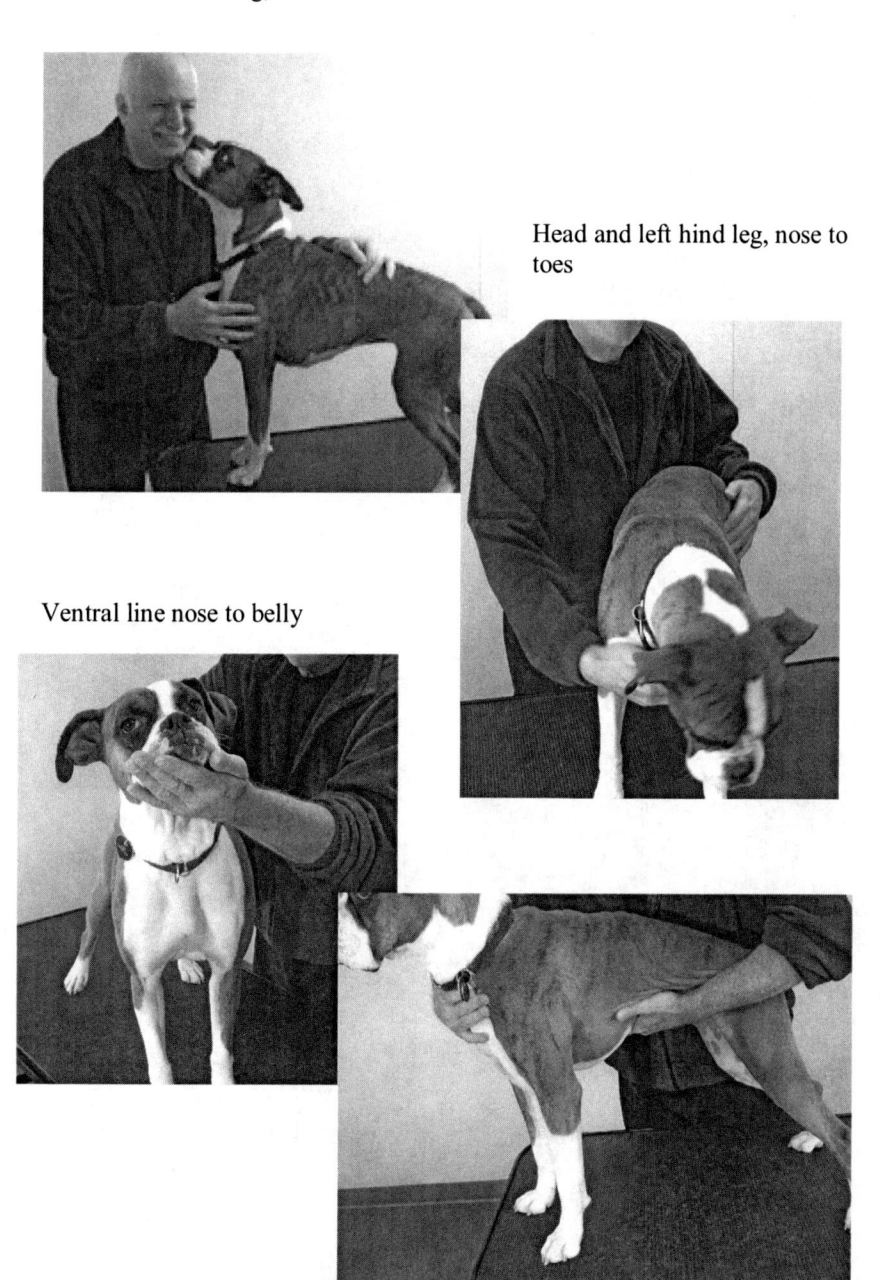

Head and left hind leg, nose to toes

Ventral line nose to belly

Head and neck
Feel for tightness and flexibility, muscle tone, tone and texture of the coat.

Frictioning

Skin rolling

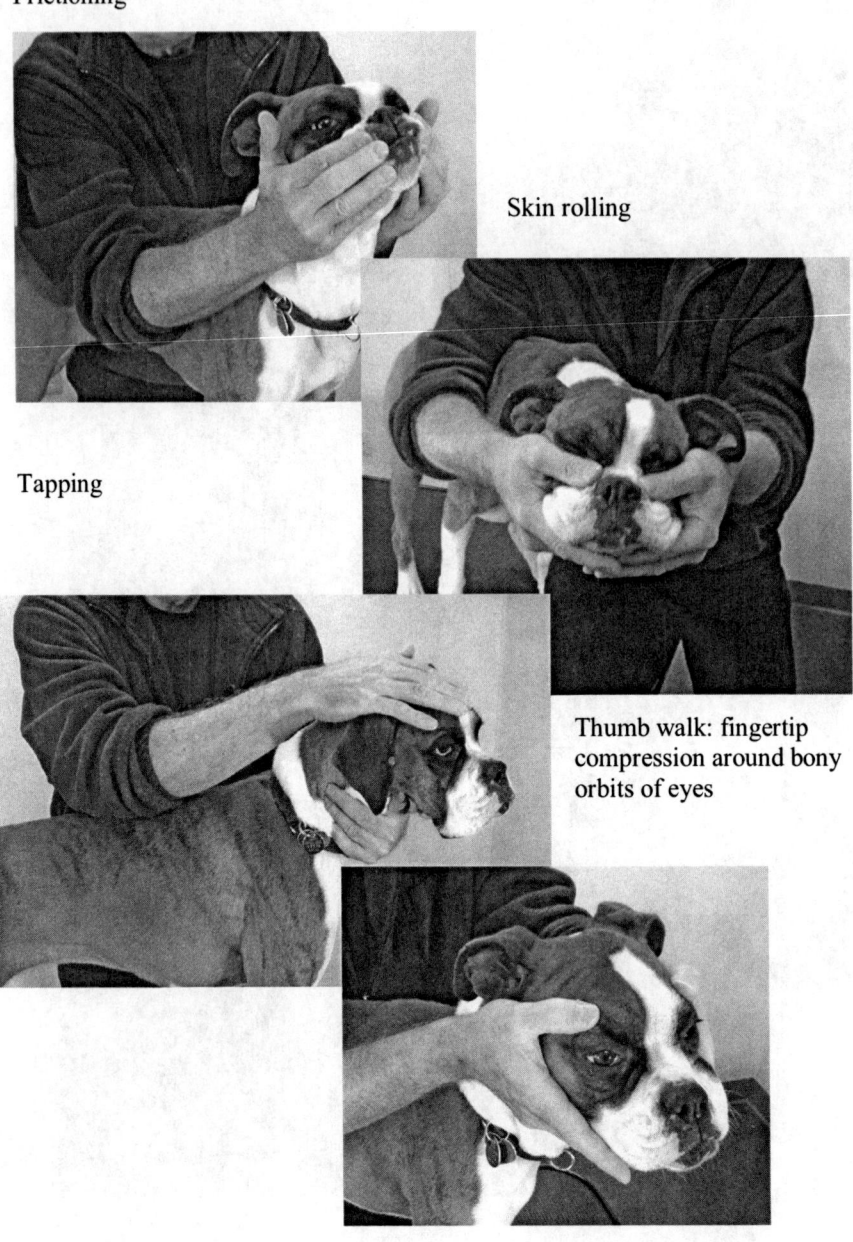

Tapping

Thumb walk: fingertip compression around bony orbits of eyes

Rocking head and neck

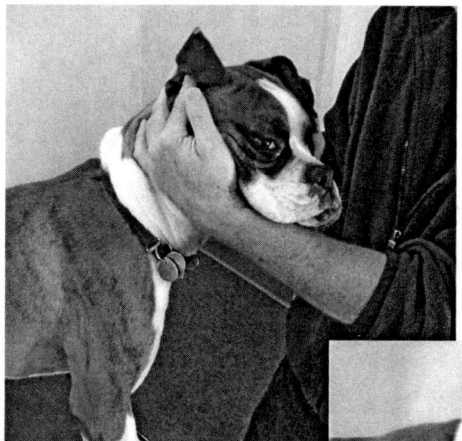

Joint mobilization of upper neck

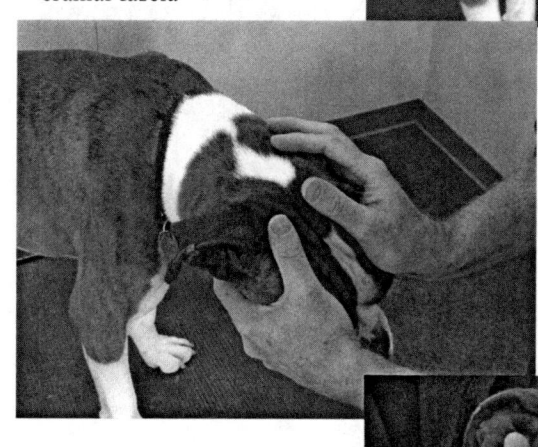

Positional release of the cranial fascia

Fingertip compression stimulating gums and stretching flew

Trunk and ribs:
All these techniques stimulate the blood and lymph circulation through the coat, skin, fascia and muscles. It also supports respiratory capacity in the fascia containing the back, neck, chest and lungs.

Skin rolling

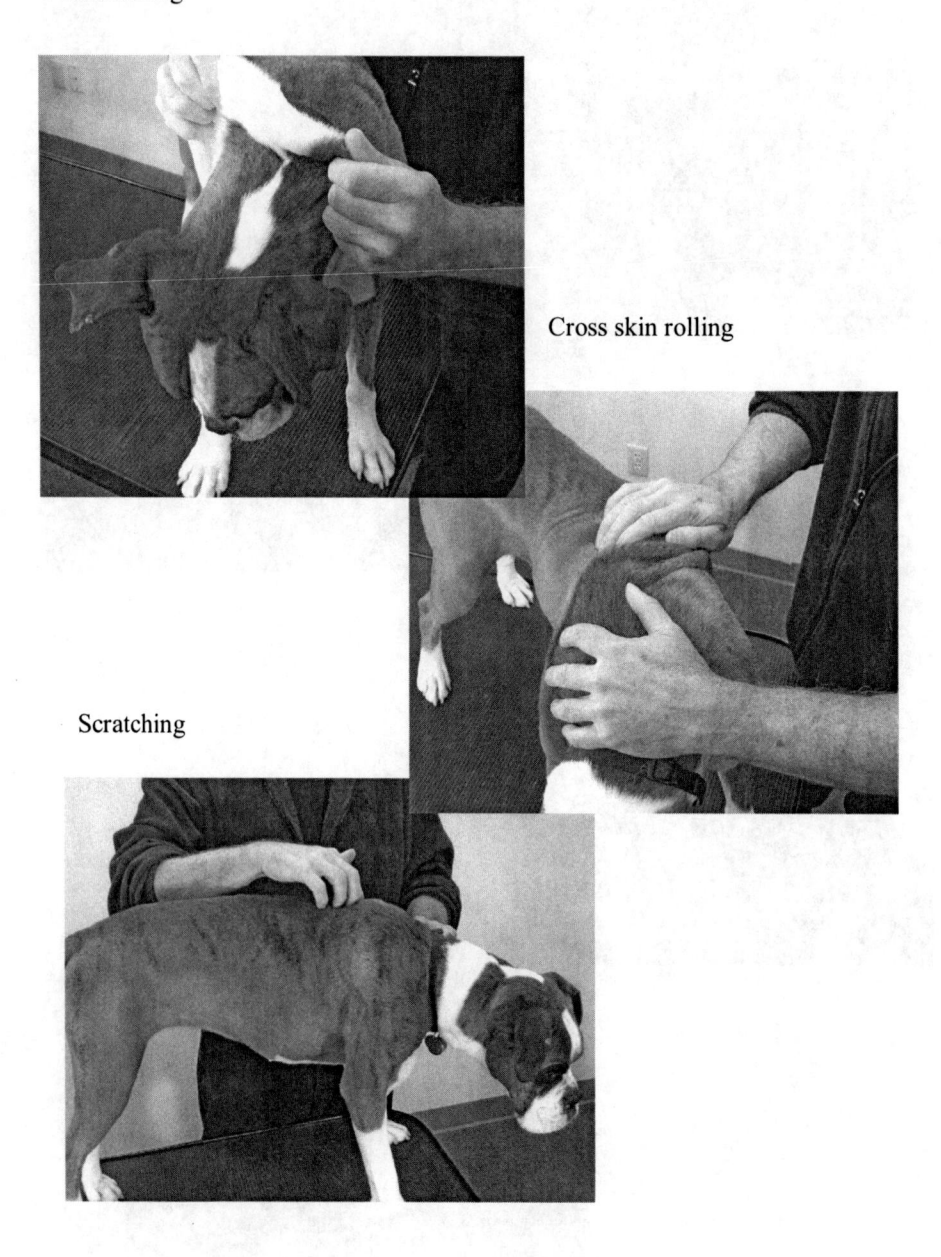

Cross skin rolling

Scratching

Clasp hands

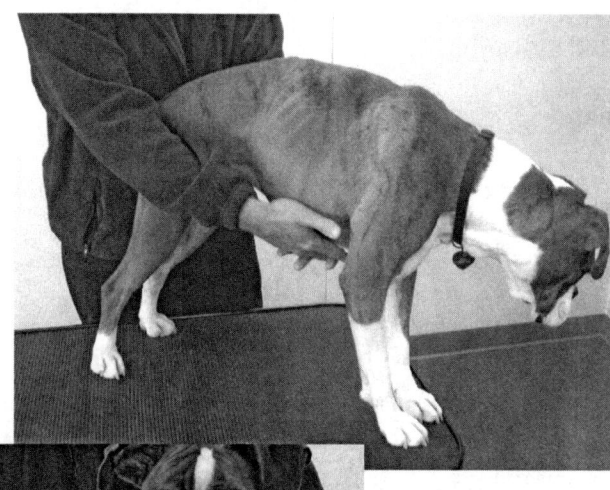

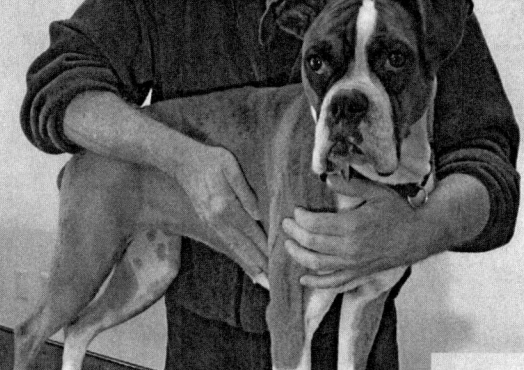

Cupping on the ribcage

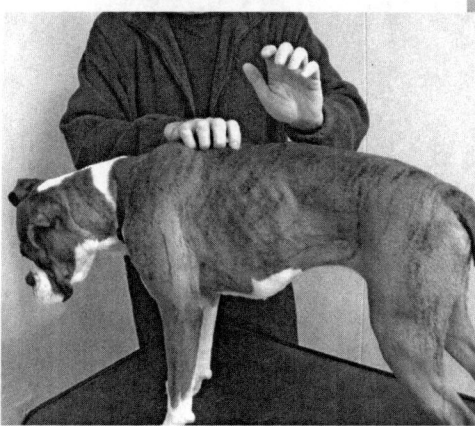

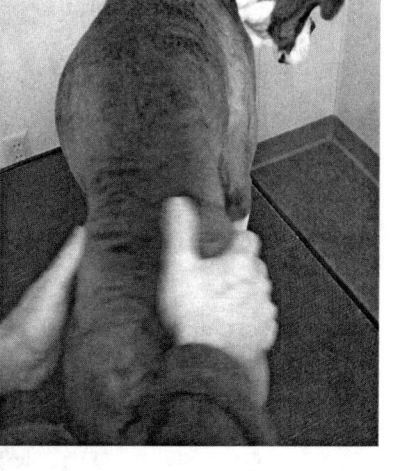

Rocking from the hips

Spinal Tapping

Legs and paws

Frictioning

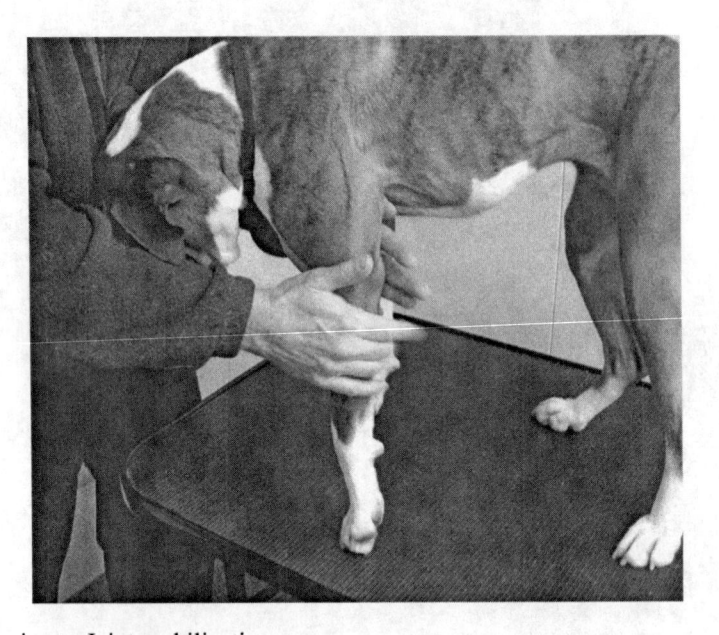

Compression to Joint mobilization

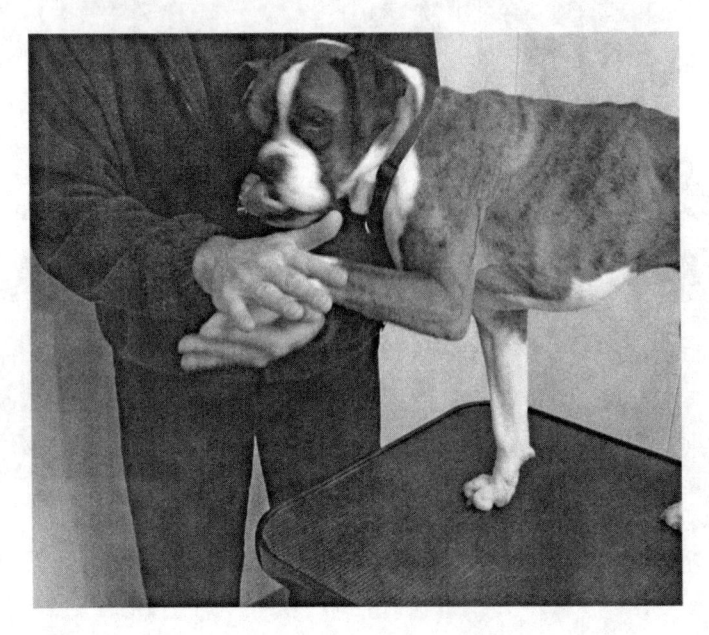

Scratching upper foreleg

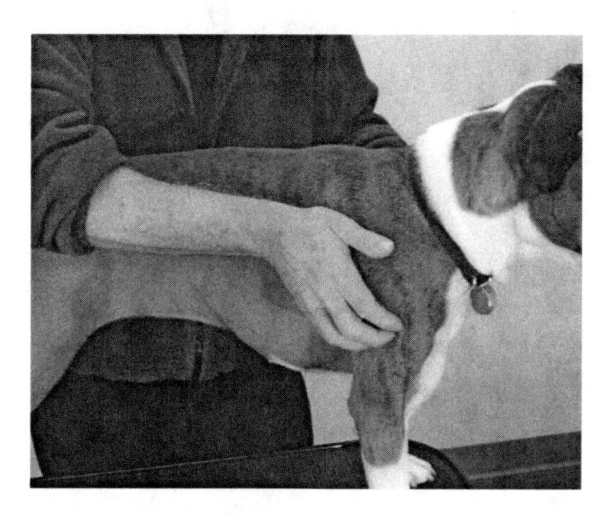

Positional release

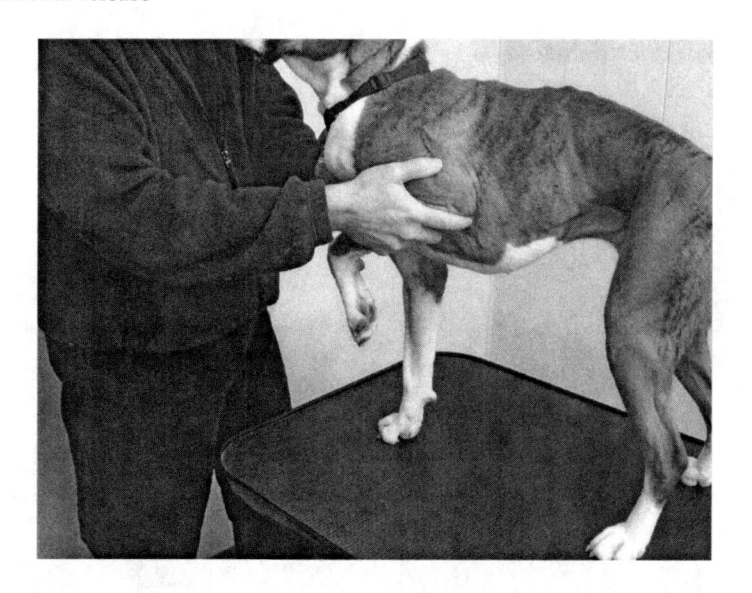

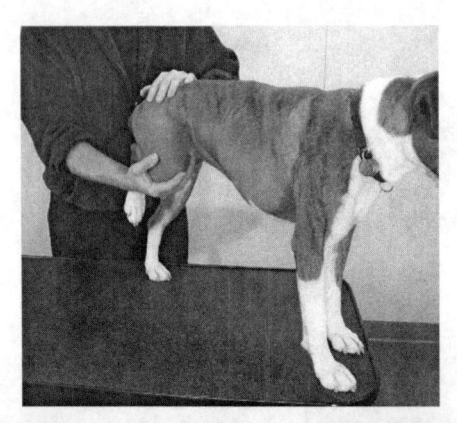

ART AND ESSENCE OF CANINE MASSAGE
PETMASSAGE™ FOR DOGS

Positional release to stretch hip

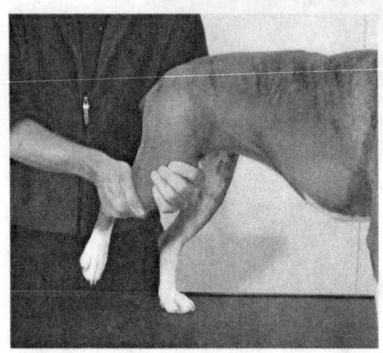

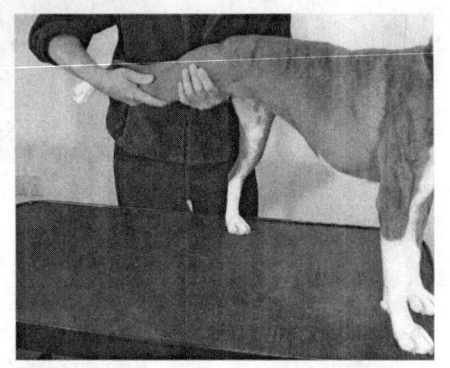

Compression to Positional release

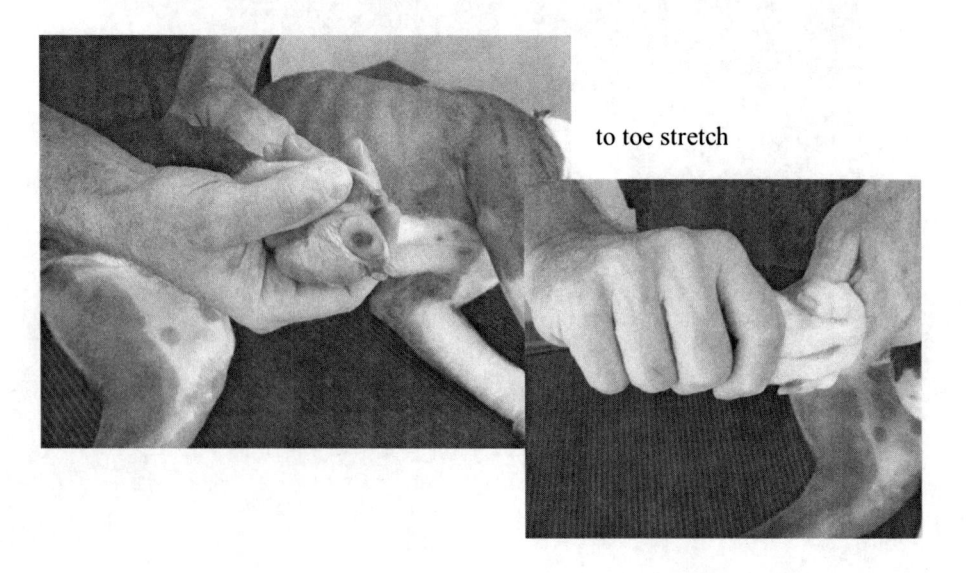

to toe stretch

Tail and lower spine

Compression

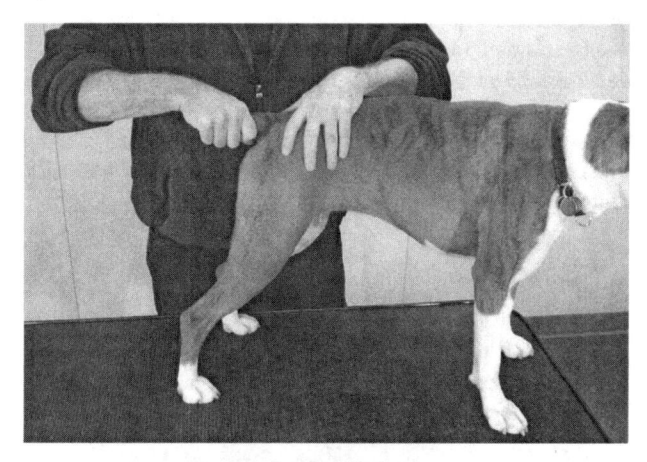

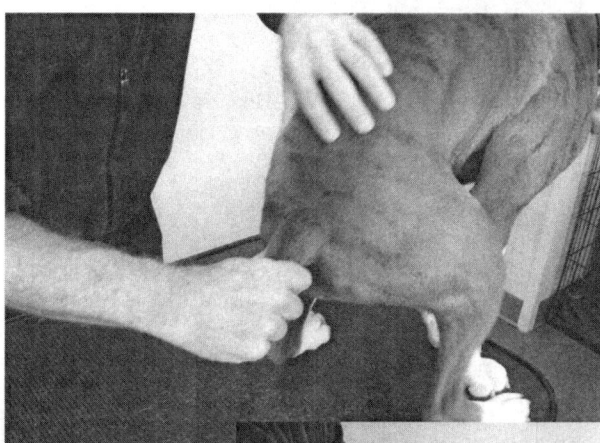

Positional release

Rocking the spine

Re-assessment strokes

Re-assess the coat, skin and superficial muscles over the six pathways of the body. Contrast any changes in texture, temperature, resilience, receptivity to first assessment stroke series.

This series is in the opposite order of depths, that is, begin with deep, then medium, and finish with light stroking. This is a signal that tells the dog that we are exiting his body space.

> Three strokes:
> 1. Deep "Here you are."
> 2. Medium "Listen to your body on this level"
> 3. Light: "Good bye, here I go. Enjoy your life."

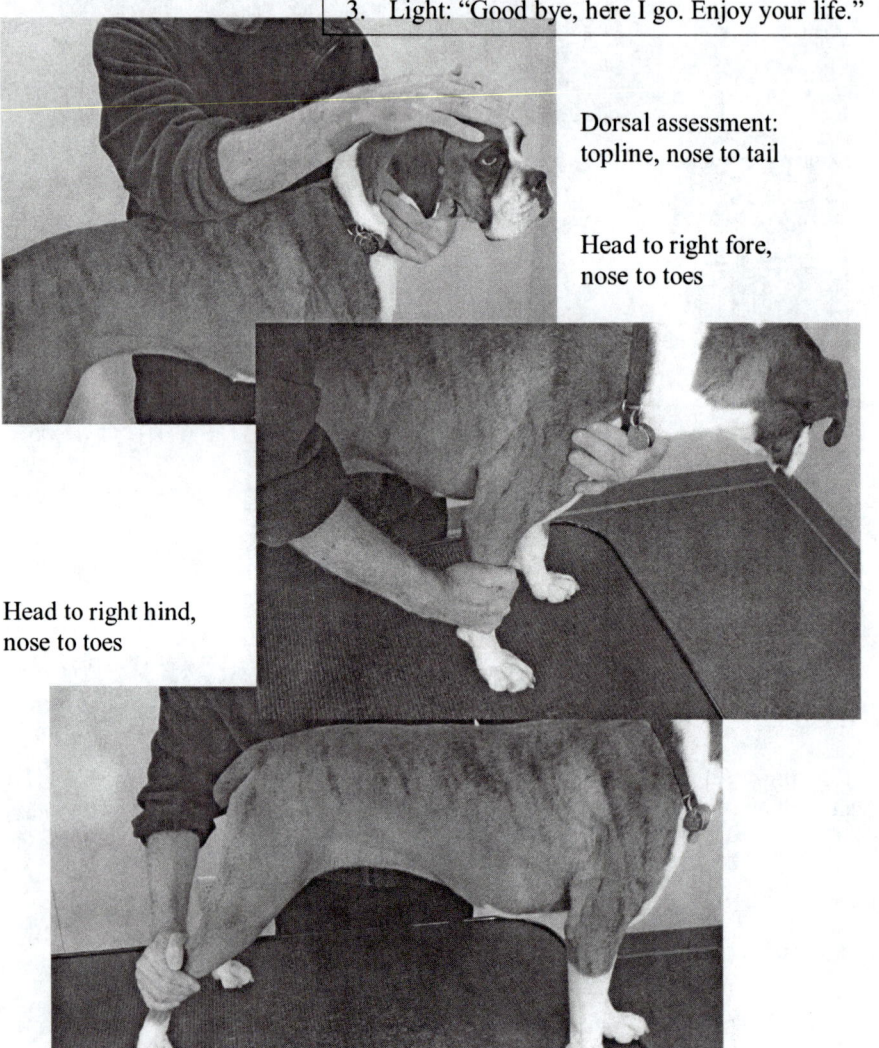

Dorsal assessment: topline, nose to tail

Head to right fore, nose to toes

Head to right hind, nose to toes

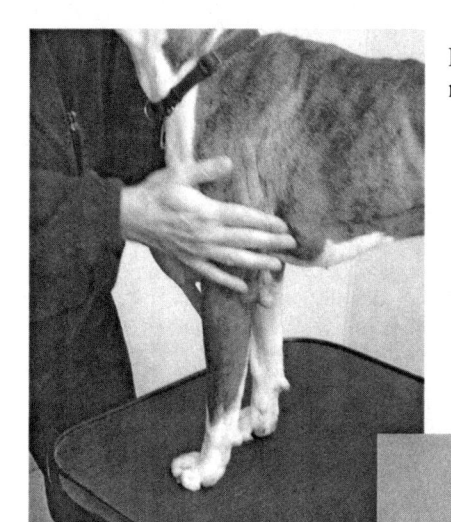

Head to left fore, nose to toes

Head to left hind, nose to toes

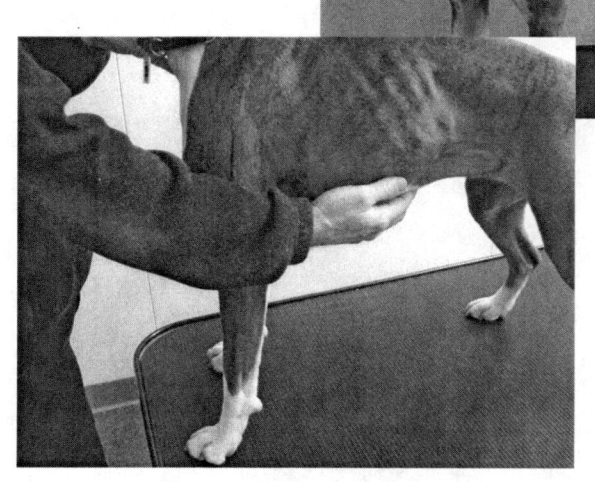

Ventral line, chin to belly

Repeat Vectoring
Begin with still-holding. Continue with your follow-on of whatever movements and shifts you observe in your bodies. Allow your hands to participate more fully in each vector's positional release. Take your time.

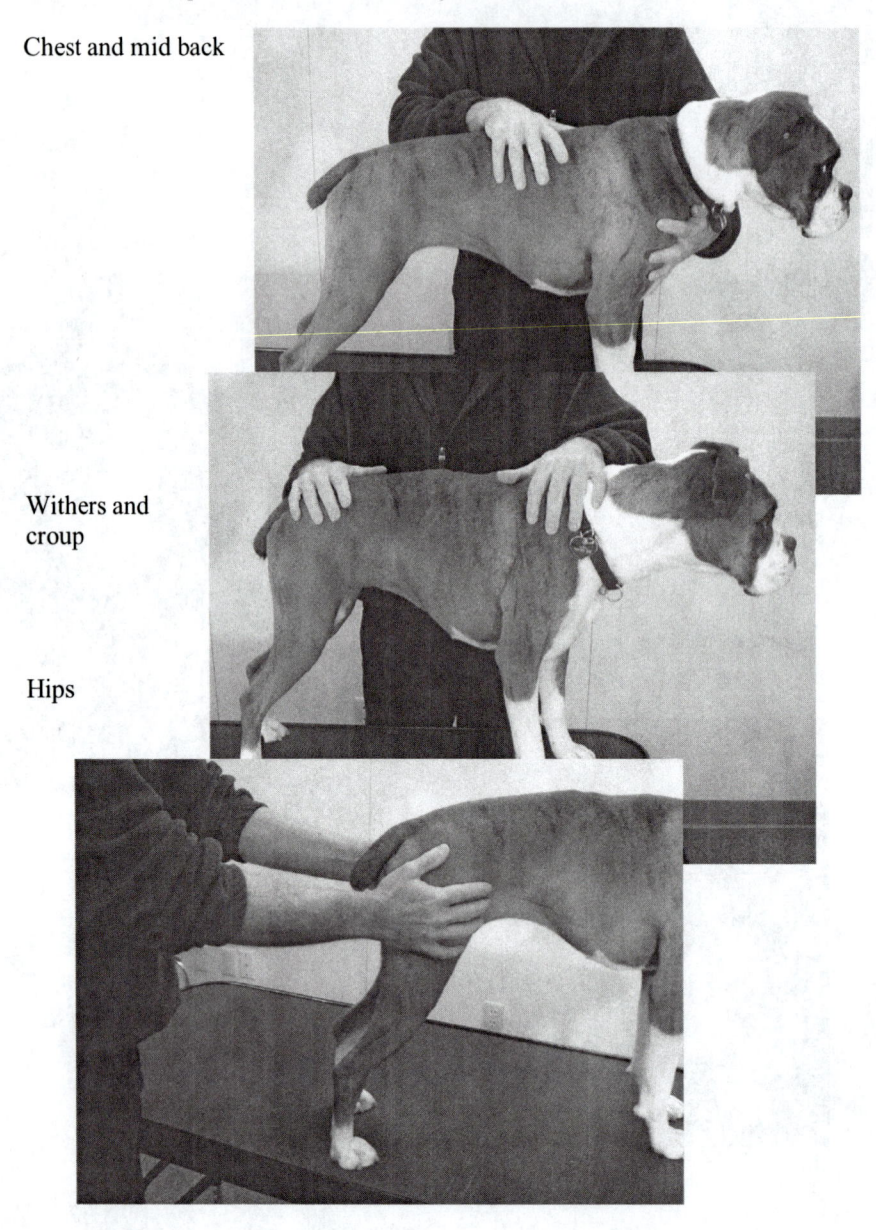

Chest and mid back

Withers and croup

Hips

Sides of ribs behind the elbows

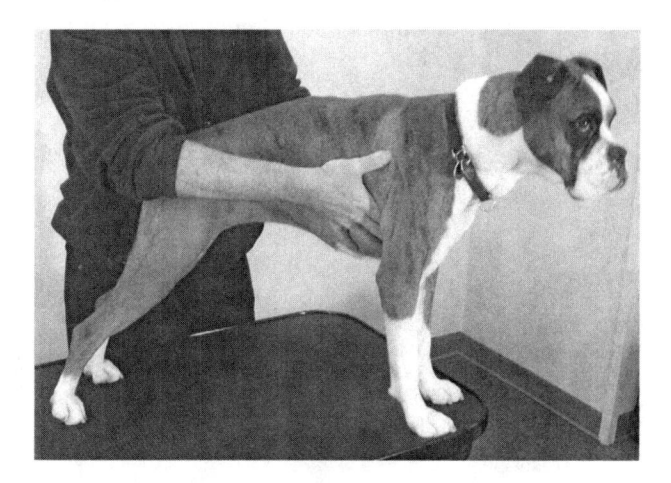

Belly and back

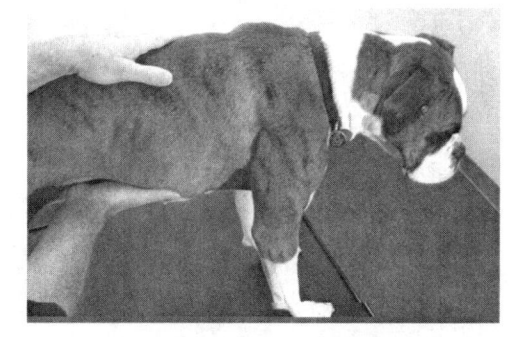

Mid back and chest

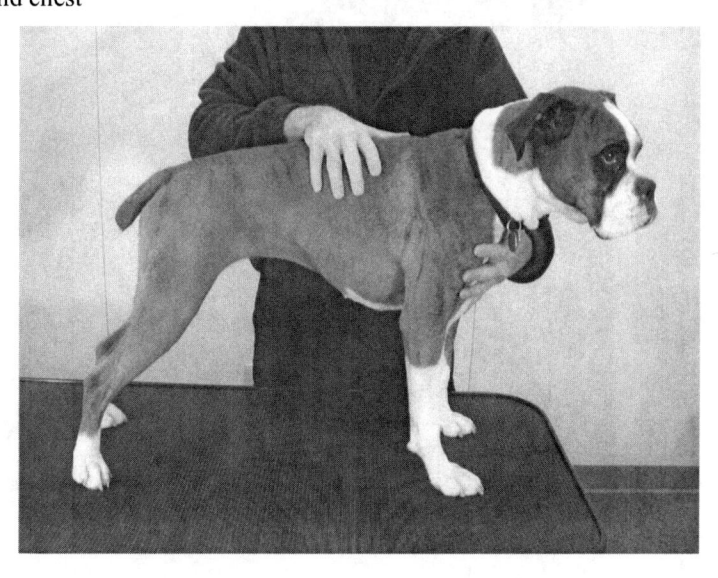

Connect the dots (both passes begin at the tail and end on the nose)
Trace a line over the ventral midline from tail to the nose.

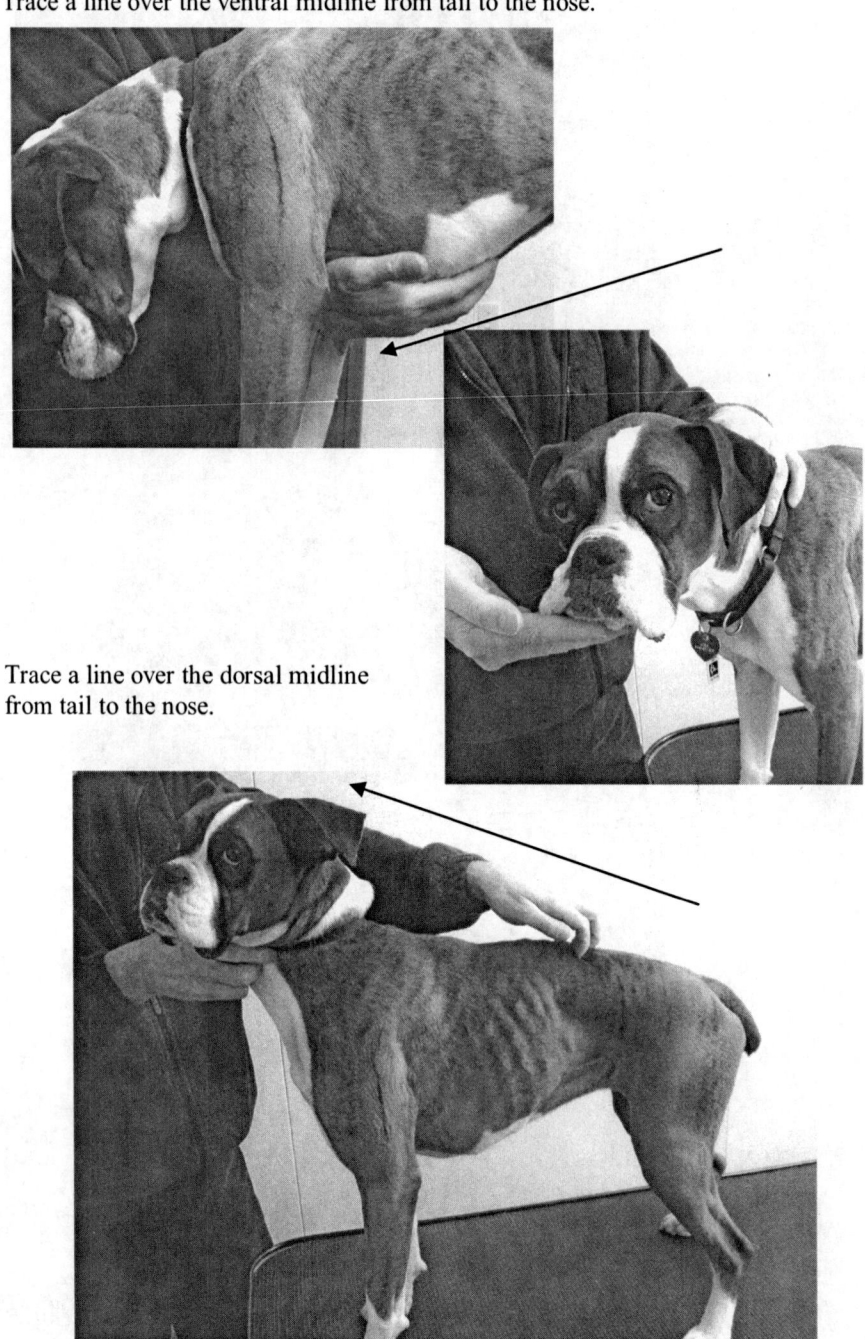

Trace a line over the dorsal midline from tail to the nose.

Grounding Cranial and Caudal

Forehand

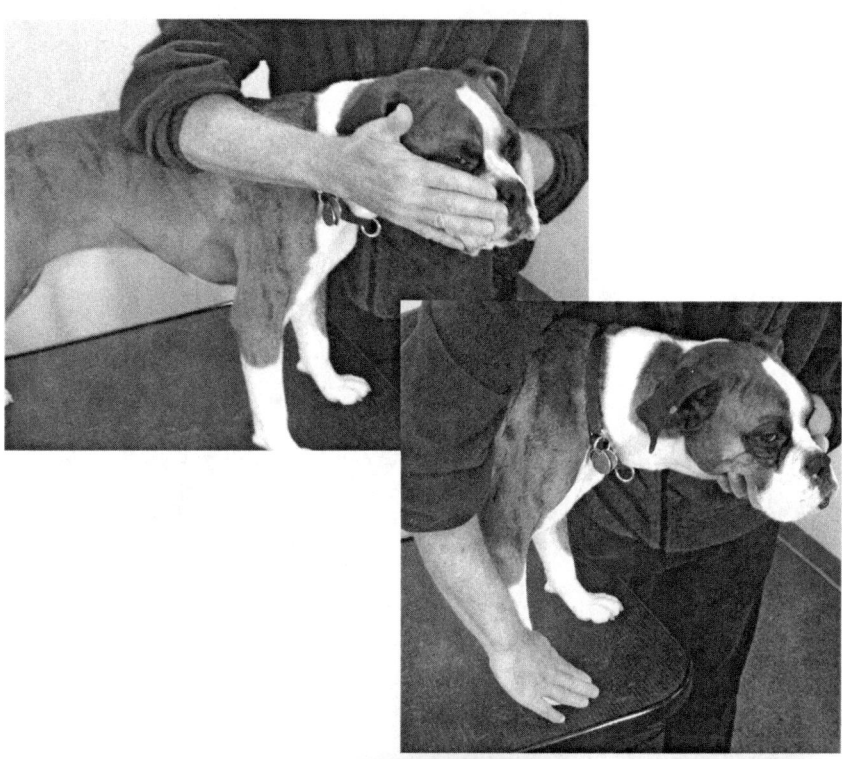

Hind limbs

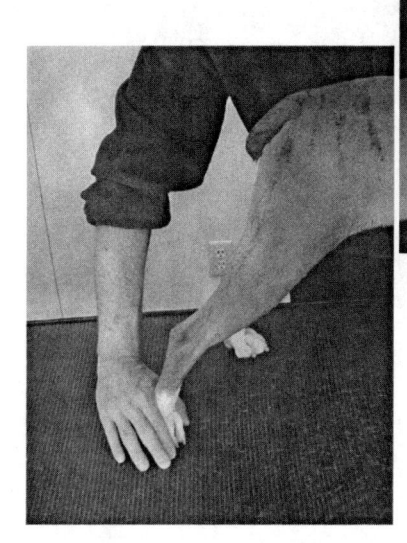

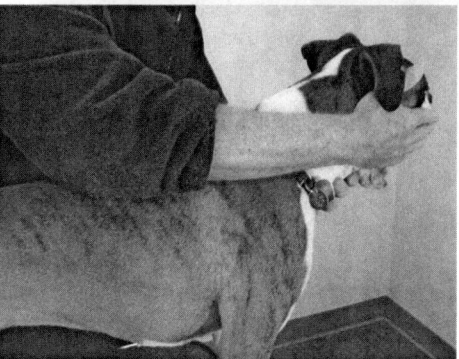

Breathing, disconnecting and thanking

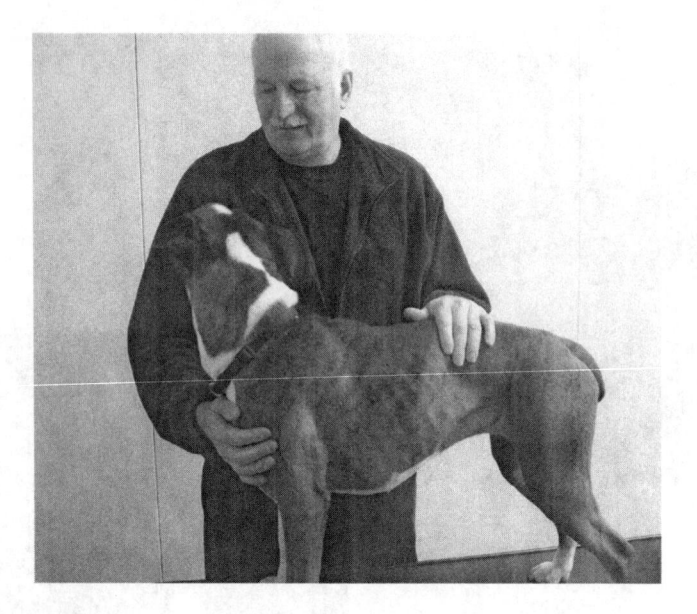

Thymus thump

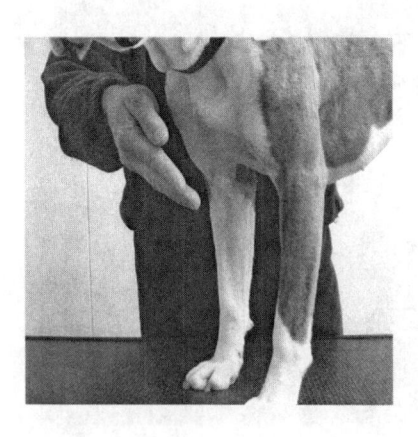

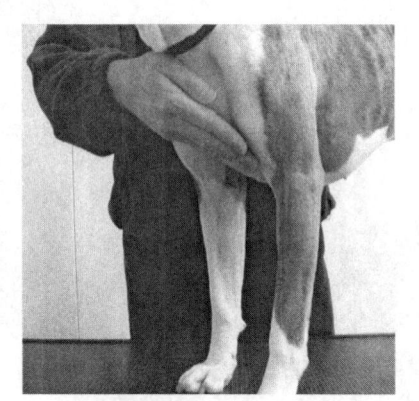

Assist dog onto floor (body mechanics)

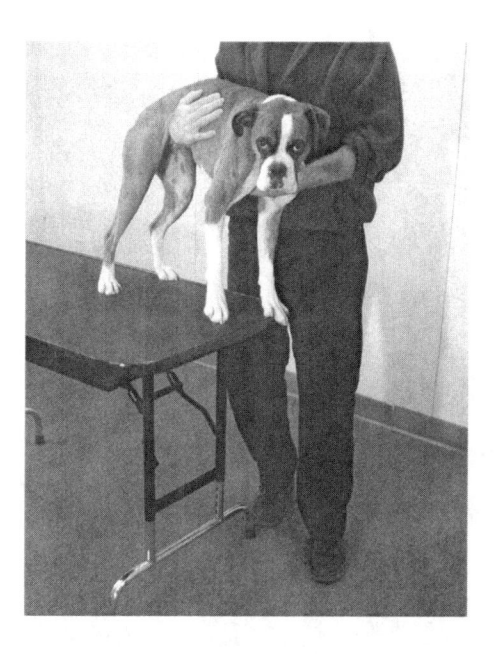

Observation of attitude, comfort, flexibility

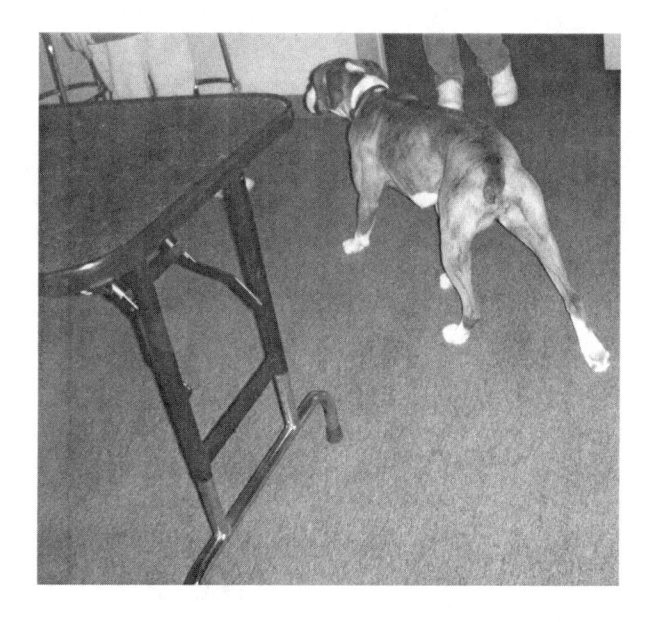

Observe gait and integration shake

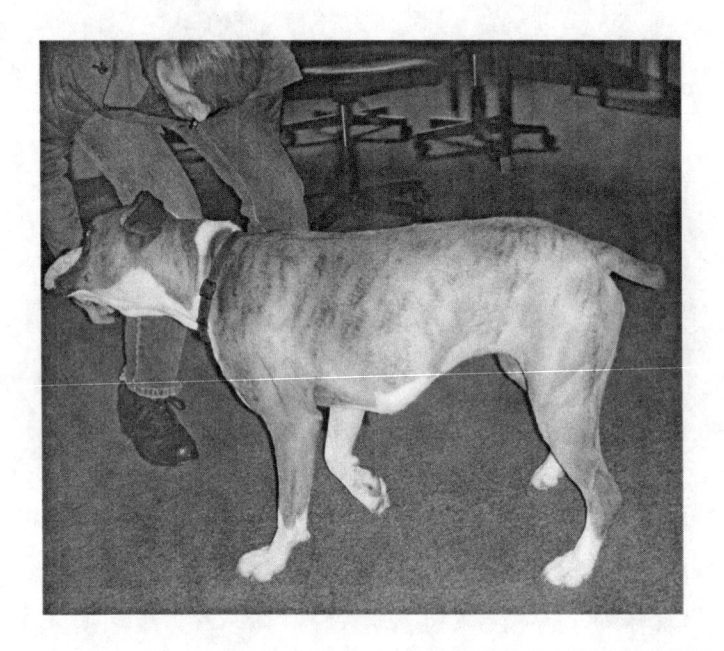

Elimination and hydration

PetMassage increases circulation, the movement of fluids in the body. All the fluids are stimulated. This includes the blood, lymph, synovial fluid in the joints, urine, fluids in the lungs and sinus cavities and moisture in the skin and hair. During a PetMassage, and for forty eight hours after it, toxins in the fascia, are released. They are released in sweat and drool. They are moved out of their cells and dumped into the blood stream, to be filtered out by the liver and kidneys, and excreted.

Your dog will need to urinate immediately after his PetMassage session. This is the reason.

This is also the rationale for offering your dog fresh water after his session. The water he takes in over the next two days will hydrate the tissues so that more toxins can flow out.

The session doesn't end for the dog when he gets off the table. You have facilitated the beginnings of additional releases, which your dog will continue to burp, fart, itch, stretch and generally unravel.

Thoughts and imaging

After you have completed the PetMassage session, and your dog is either resting quietly back on the floor or has left with his guardian, sit quietly and review what has just occurred. Replay in your mind as much of the session as you can remember. Your review of the high points, and your visceral reaction to them will continue to strengthen the new dog's connections.

At this time, you may be able to access and release, in your mind's eye, areas that you were either unable to get to or ones that hadn't attracted your attention during the physical session.

If the dog is still in discomfort, or is in the process of his continuing rehabilitation or treatment, see him as whole and healthy. Visualize him in an open field, in the sunshine, running and jumping and playing.

This meditation may take a few minutes or several. The breathing exercise on page 64 is also helpful for closure. Any breathwork you do, supports both you and your dog.

Documentation

Good and responsible record keeping is essential to establishing and maintaining professionalism in your work. Your record keeping has various functions, such as organizing and managing your schedule, communicating with other members of your dog's wellness team, and sending and receiving documents.

The quality of records you keep will be the basis for keeping track of your clients. The upper part of the form on the following pages provides you with valuable marketing information such as the preferred way they would like to be contacted, their email address, and the dog's birth date.

Your notes will also be helpful when your clients return for additional sessions. Reviewing notes of what you had done previously will give you an idea of what to expect.

Many of the dogs who are brought to you for PetMassage will be seeking your services for specific reasons. True, some are receiving the equivalent of a spa treatment, for relaxation and pampering; however, most are dealing with a specific physical or behavioral "issue." These dogs are in training for competition, or are on weight loss regimens; they have chronic health conditions, or are at the end stages of life. Some of them are under veterinary supervised rehabilitation programs.

Your sessions and contributions need to be tracked. Your written impressions can be of enormous help to the pet's guardians and staffs of their veterinary clinics. Your notes document how the dog is progressing, staying the same, or regressing. You and your colleagues need to know what role PetMassage has in the dog's wellness care and recovery.

The most often used form for describing a session are the S.O.A.P. notes. SOAP stands for
- Subjective, what you perceive
- Objective, what you measure
- Action, what you do
- Plan, what you encourage your dog to do

Narrative notes may be easier for you. They will have similar information as in the SOAP notes, but you can write them as a paragraph. Use your own words to describe your dog's life condition, what was successful or unsuccessful in your session, what were your dog's responses and reactions to various types of skill applications and pressures, what follow up measures do you plan to take, such as phoning, emailing, scheduling future sessions, or instructions for the guardian to continuing maintenance. [Borcherding]

The BIRP form is also good for canine PetMassage. BIRP stands for
- B: The behavior that is exhibited by the dog
- I: The PetMassage (intervention)
- R: The dog's response to the PetMassage
- P: Your plan for continued intervention, based on the dog's response

The PIRP is another. It stands for
- P: The problem or purpose of the PetMassage treatment
- IRP: The intervention, response and plan

If there is ever a legal challenge to the way a dog has been treated, your notes can be subpoenaed, as legal documents, along with those of veterinarians, as part of the dog's health history. Your records must be clear, easy to maintain, and available, if necessary. There are some basic standards for legal documents to be admissible in court. They must be written, not printed, in blue or black ink, not pencil. There can be no erasures; so, if you misspell a word or change your mind about a phrase or term, you must draw a line (only one line--do not crosshatch or scribble over your mistake) through the words you want to delete, initial the change, and write the words you want.

The following is a "boiler plate" version for your intake form and records. Please adapt it as you choose. One month after the photo of the Bernese Mountain Dog puppy was taken, she looked very different. Requesting a current photo is a good reason to contact past clients. In documentation, the term "lesson" may be used when references to a manual therapy "session" of animals is restricted.

ART AND ESSENCE OF CANINE MASSAGE
PETMASSAGE™ FOR DOGS

Example
Intake form

Dog's Name_____

Your company name　　　　　　　Date_____
Your address
City, State, Zip
Phone
Email

Dog's Name_____

Breed _____ Age ____ Birth date _____

Description _____

Sensitive areas/ unique qualities _____
_____
_____

Complaint _____
_____

Previous Treatments _____

Veterinarian_____ Phone _____

Name of Caregiver _____

Address _____

City _____ ST ____ Zip _____

Phone (cell) _____ Phone (home/work) _____

Email _____

First photo of dog　　　　　　　　Two months later

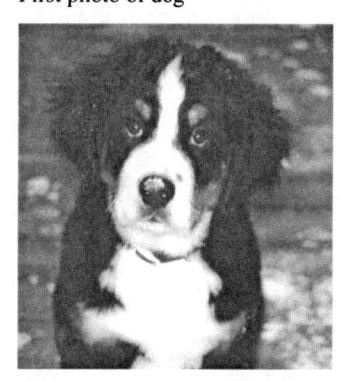

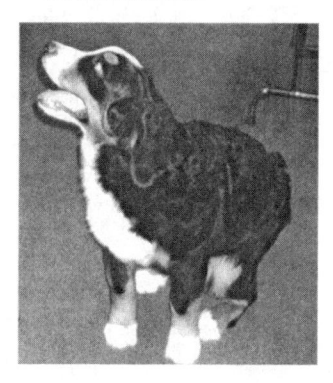

ART AND ESSENCE OF CANINE MASSAGE
PETMASSAGE™ FOR DOGS

Session/Lesson 1
_____
_____
_____

Session/Lesson 2
_____
_____
_____

Session/Lesson 3
_____
_____
_____

Session/Lesson 4
_____
_____
_____

Session/Lesson 5
_____
_____
_____

Clients can sign or initial a consent form, stating that they understand that you cannot diagnose, prescribe medications, or be held responsible for any injuries that may result from the owners practicing massage techniques on their own dogs.

Suggested Disclaimer:
Massage is not, nor is it intended to be a substitute for traditional veterinary care. It is a complementary form of health care. The pet guardian should regularly consult a veterinarian in matters relating to his or her dog's health and especially in regard to any symptoms, which may require diagnosis or medical attention. If you have any questions regarding the efficacy of any of the techniques provided, please consult with your veterinarian or qualified PetMassage practitioner.

Working with any animal involves inherent risk. While general PetMassage techniques are all applied lovingly and gently, any receiver, animal or human, may react negatively to strokes they may perceive as abusive, invasive, or inappropriate.

I have read and understand this disclaimer.

Signed and dated _____

Benefits for dogs

PetMassage and bodywork may be the only way to address many of the holding patterns muscle groups have developed. PetMassage enables your dog's body, mind and spirit to relax and fine tune his life condition.

Here are some of the many benefits for dogs.

- #1 Reason: Enhances quality of life
- PetMassage helps dogs maintain and restore flexibility, ROM (range of motion) and ROE (range of emotion).
- It increases or balances circulation of blood, lymph, CSF (cerebral-spinal fluid), oxygen, awareness and Chi.
- Strengthens the body by stimulating muscles
- Increases muscle tone and use
- PetMassage helps your dog develop trust. He learns to accept, appreciate and encourage touch, especially to his paws.
- Provides comfort to tired muscles and often induces relief from pain
- PetMassage helps with bonding. Dogs will be more comfortable in his people's presence, as they become more aware of their body language.
- It energizes the dog's mind.
- It increases the dog's sense of self, body awareness.
- Supports health and wellness in every stage of dogs' lives

Geriatric PetMassage session

The population that could use all the benefits PetMassage offers the most are the seniors. As these dogs slow down, and exercise less, their faculties to fight discomfort and disease diminishes. Aging is the natural cycle of slowing down, stiffness, guarding from pain, degeneration, atrophy, despair, disease and eventually, death. *PetMassage can intervene at every one of these stages. It can help the dog to attain a better quality of life with less pain, more body awareness and a sense of control.* PetMassage enhances dogs' immune systems by increasing cardiovascular circulation. It increases flexibility in joints, promotes muscle tone and supports neural/brain activity. Combine all these benefits with special one-on-one time and you have a very happy and appreciative canine!

The elements and order for a geriatric PetMassage session.
- Observation of gait, comportment
- Situating the dog onto the table
- Permission
- Vectoring
- Assessment strokes
- Skin rolling and compression to joint mobilization on major joints
- Positional release to stretching of all major joints and fascia Scratching up and down spine and over major lymph nodes
- Clasp hands and cupping on ribcage
- Rocking the body, side-lying or standing
- Jostle the limbs and tail
- Assessment repeat
- Vector repeat
- Connect the dots and Ground
- Thump and thank
- Assist dog from table to floor and observe integration shake and gait
- Elimination and hydration

Sports PetMassage

Warm up

Warm your dog's tissues before competitions and heavy exertion. He will move faster, smoother, and more balanced. He'll also have less chance of injuring his body.

Warm the muscles, or soft tissue, *before* stretching. Stretching is not the same as warm up; it is just a part of it. In your enthusiasm use caution so that you do not hyperextend any of the joints without first warming them.

Use friction, muscle compression, and joint manipulation over the major joints, working forward from the base of the tail to the skull, and upward from each of the legs from the paws to the topline. Your movements are intended to stimulate, so they move against the lay of the coat.

Warm up movements are faster and more rigorous than a standard PetMassage. You know the tissues are warming when your hands feel hot.

- Assist dog onto PetMassage table
- Get dog's permission
- Center yourself and the dog
- Vector
- Apply progressively rapid assessment strokes to increase dog's body awareness and body excitement.
- Warm the entire body with frictioning and skin rolling.
- Stay within the dog's normal ROM. All hyperextensions will be unwindings from the dog, as positional release follow-on's.

- Work the major joints and large muscle groups starting with the head and neck, and working the shoulders, forelegs, spine employing skin rolling, joint manipulation and tapotement,
rolling and rocking, scratching, clasp hands and cupping
- On the hips and hamstrings: stimulate the groove up the back of each of the rear legs from the back of the stifle to the sit bone (ischial tuberosity)
- Frictioning, compression, joint mobilization to stretching the paws and digits
- On the tail apply gentle traction, pulling in small circles, finishing with positional release of the tail and spine
- Scratch up and down the body, neck and legs with big sweeping motions from caudal to cranial, against the lay of he hair, to increase the circulation throughout the body. Scratch with medium to deep pressure.
- Complete with vectoring
- Grounding
- Thymus thump
- Assist dog from table onto the ground
- Observe gait and integration shake
- Elimination and hydration

Cool down

After an event, or extreme exertion, a cool down PetMassage will encourage fatigued or strained muscle tissue to have a quick recovery. Its function is to increase the cardiovascular circulation and drain the lymph nodes while slowing the respiratory rate.

The post event cool down naturally clears away the toxic chemicals that have been released by the body.

- Assist dog onto PetMassage table
- Get dog's permission.
- Breathe with the dog, to center yourself and the dog.
- Vector
- Assessment strokes, progressively slowing, to calm the dog's excitement.
- Rhythmic medium to light scratching over the entire body from cranial to caudal and midline towards the extremities.
- Gently rock and jostle the major joints and spine.
- Positional release of the paws, with compression to joint manipulation on each digit (remember to include the dewclaw, or its scar).
- Final assessment strokes in the order of deep, medium and light.
- Vector sequence using positional release
- Ground, smoothing the surface of the body with slow, graceful hand sweeping motions from head to tail and from nose to toes on all four legs.
- Still-hold the dog and breathe rhythmically
- Thymus thump
- Assist dog from table onto the ground
- Observe integration shake and gait
- Elimination and hydration

PetMassage focus on the tail

PetMassage tail work has many benefits.

- It increases circulation and flexibility to the joints and tissues
- Enhances circulation and flexibility to the dorsal and ventral aspects of the entire spine
- Enhances circulation and flexibility to the lateral oblique muscles
- Enhances the activities and function of the central nervous system running through the spine
- Supports the dog's ability to communicate with other dogs
- Supports the dog's balance and flexibility while running and turning
- Initiates a weight bearing exercise, as the dog catches her weight, side to side
- Increases bone density

The canine tail usually consists of between six and 23 highly mobile vertebrae. These vertebrae are enclosed by a versatile musculature that make the various segments, especially the tip, capable of highly controlled movements that lift the tail, move it from side to side, or draw it down toward the anus or between the hind legs.

Dogs use their tails for communicating. They express happiness, aggression, stress and many other emotions with their tail. By looking at the position and movement of the tail, you can often tell what dogs are thinking. When a dog wags his tail high and wags it back and forth, he's usually feeling pretty good. When he is interested in something, his tail is usually horizontal to the ground. A tucked tail indicates the dog is frightened or submissive. When the tail goes from horizontal to upright and becomes rigid, he is feeling threatened or challenged. A low and wagging tail indicates the dog is worried or insecure.

The tail is used to communicate with other animals. Every time your dog moves his tail, it acts like a perfume atomizer and spreads his natural scent around him. One of his most important odors comes from the anal glands, two sacs under the tail that contain an odiferous liquid that is as unique among dogs as fingerprints are to us. Every time the dog wags his tail, the muscles around the anus contract and press on the glands, causing a release of the scent. A dominant dog that carries his tail high releases much more scent than a dog that holds his tail lower. Likewise, a frightened dog holds his tail between his legs to keep others from sniffing him, and in that way makes himself invisible, in an aromatic world.

The tail is important as a means of counterbalance when the dog is carrying out complicated movements such as leaping, walking along narrow structures or climbing. Sight hounds that run at great speeds often have thin tails that are very long in proportion to the rest of their body. They use their tails as a counterbalance when making turns. Their tails may increase their agility and ability to turn quickly, so they can keep up with their prey. Tail muscles are also important in stabilizing the vertebral column and supporting the action of the extensor muscles of the back, as well as those of the croup and buttocks.

Some dogs use their tails as rudders when swimming. Dogs bred for swimming frequently have tails that are thick, strong and very flexible, which helps them to move easily through the water and make quick turns.

Some dogs use their tails for insulation. Nordic and Arctic breeds have bushy or plumed tails with long dense fur. When lying down they may pull their tails over their faces to keep out the cold. They also use their tails as rudders when pulling a sled across the ice. [Wells]

The hand position you use depends on the natural curl of the tail. With most dogs, your palm will be turned down. With dogs whose tail curl naturally over their backs, your palms will be up.

PetMassage of the tail includes frictioning, using both hands to warm the tissues and joint mobilization, and using one hand in a muscle squeezing/wringing motion to each of the joints of the tail. Make sure that your mother hand is in contact with the dog at all times. When you lift both of your hands off the body, dogs read this as a disconnect and a signal that the session is over.

If you notice any tightness or stiffness, this can often be resolved with positional release, working with two to five joint segments at a time.

The base of the tail is an extension of the myofascial tissue running the full length of the spine and onto the top of the head. Supporting the tail set, lift the tail so that it is a continuation of the curve of the croup, extending caudally from the spine. Maintain a gentle traction (light pressure) to the tail, and move the group of tail vertebrae closest to the sacrum in slow, small circles, first in one direction, then the other. This effectively warms and stimulates the muscles, tendons and ligaments that attach around the anus, to the pelvic girdle, and to the lower spine.

Apply positional release to the tail so that it adjusts its relationship to the spine. Continuing to grasp the tail, applying steady gentle traction. Rock your body from side to side, encouraging a similar movement in the dog's body. The progressively vigorous movement will eventually have the dog's body flexing from side to side as he transfers his weight to maintain balance.

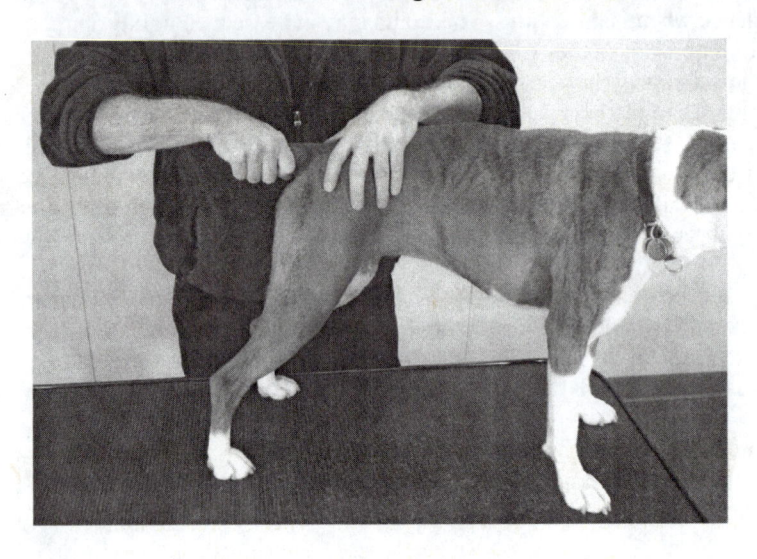

PetMassage focus on the neck

Dogs show very similar head postures as humans and appear to communicate similar emotional states. When they are happy, they raise their heads. When they are sad, they hang their heads, with the dorsal muscles supporting the weight. When they question, they cock their head to one side. When they are expressing dominance, they arch their necks so they can look down on their subordinates from a position of power. When expressing submission, they lower their chins so that they are looking up.

Dogs necks also carry similar human-type emotional based stresses and strains. PetMassage of the neck helps dogs with stiff necks. Obese dogs often have folds of fat hindering their full range of movement and have difficulty turning their heads. This lack of movement puts stress on the body. Reduced circulation of blood and lymph as well as of other fluids to and from the skull, cause a reduced sense of balance.

The dog's neck is an interesting part of its anatomy. There is a large mass of muscle tissue which encases and protects the important spinal cord, larynx and esophagus. The muscles and fascial connections provide movement and support to the head, neck, shoulders, and upper arms. There are muscles that originate on the vertebral column and insert on the skull. There are muscles with both their origin and insertion on the vertebral column. There are muscles originating on the shoulder girdle and inserting on the skull. There are muscles originating on the vertebral column and inserting on the shoulder girdle; and muscles originating on the rib cage and inserting on the vertebral column. There are ventral muscles and sub-occipital muscles. [Sharir]

Deep within these muscles are the seven cervical vertebrae which connect the base of the skull, at the foramen magnum, to the thoracic vertebrae.

The vertebrae give structure to the neck and provide safe passage for the central nervous system. The two upper most bones, the atlas and the axis, are palpable at the base of the skull. The middle four vertebrae are deep within the musculature. And the seventh vertebra is accessible when it emerges between the wings of the scapula.

With all these muscles interweaving amongst each other it can be daunting to attempt to stimulate or relax one group while not disturbing another. PetMassage simplifies the process. The PetMassage experience generally balances the tissues, increasing circulation where it needs it, and inducing flexibility where there is stiffness. PetMassage approaches the neck from various angles and with various techniques, engaging the inner dog to frame his own shifts in realignment.

Skin rolling with twisting is a great way to increase circulation and induce the tissues to heat up. Rocking and joint mobilization of the upper neck and head increases flexibility. Positional release increases the circulation and flexibility to a neck that is holding the pattern of immobility, whether it is from stress, old age or obesity. A golden retriever that was grieving the loss of her canine companion of many years, had a physical/emotional release when I supported under her chin with my mother hand and applied very light touch to the back of the base of her skull with my active hand. In as little as five seconds, she was able to let go and move on with her life.

Approach with positional release on dogs heads in various angles. Dogs spontaneously move into their exploration of movement as they search for and discover new and more comfortable ways of holding their heads.

PetMassage focus on the shoulder

The canine shoulder joint is the least stable joint in the body, relying completely on soft tissue structures for stability. Stress is placed on the shoulder through hard playing, turning quickly, and giving too many high fives. Clinical signs of shoulder imbalances can range from refusing tight turns to dogs with intermittent to persistent unilateral forelimb lameness. Gait analysis ranges from a mildly shortened stride in the affected forelimb at a walk and a trot to a significant weight-bearing lameness. When abducting the shoulder, spasm and discomfort are almost always noted. [VOSM]

The components of the shoulder include the joint capsule, medial gleno-humeral ligament, the subscapularis tendon, the supraspinatus and the biceps tendons. The point of the shoulder is the joint of the upper arm that connects the humerus to the scapula. Muscle groups that attach on the trunk of the dog move through the shoulder and insert on the arm. It is important to remember that the fascia that groups the muscles, tendons and ligaments in the lower arm are all part of a larger fascia bundle that communicates with the shoulder, neck, and head.

PetMassage of the shoulder begins with frictioning to warm tissues. Place one hand in the axilla, arm pit, with palm facing out and the other cupped over the deltoid muscle on the upper arm. Press and release, gently pumping the tissues with both hands, using medium to deep pressure. Continue your compression with both hands supporting the shoulder and both alternatively acting as the Mother and the active, to increase flexibility.

Without sliding across the surface of the coat, press the skin so that it is moving across the underlying structures (bones, muscles, etc.).

Continue joint mobilization, pressing your palms toward each other and moving the tissues between them in small circles first in one direction, then the other. Expand the movement by shifting your axilla hand to support the leg just above the elbow. Assist the upper arm into slightly larger circles, staying well within the limits of the dog's comfort and range of motion. Apply positional release, observing the follow-on and when appropriate, guiding the upper arm into a gentle stretch. The foreleg always stretches forward and down; never to the side.

Continue by quieting your movement, slowly coming to a rest. Still-hold the shoulder within your hands. Breathe. Apply positional release again, observe and participate in the follow-on.

This routine increases circulation to the arm and shoulder, increases flexibility and range of motion to the shoulder. Light scratching over the axilla and across the scapula, both in the direction of the heart stimulates the axillary lymph nodes, and encourages lymphatic fluid drainage. And finally, it supports the nervous system opening pathways for cranial nerves.

PetMassage focus on the hip

The hip is one of the most vulnerable joints in the dog's body. The hip joint is a "ball and socket" type joint attaching the rear leg to the trunk of the body. The "ball" part is the head of the first long bone of the rear leg – the femur – and the socket is the part of the pelvis known as the acetabulum. The acetabulum is formed by the juncture of all three bones of the pelvis, the ilium, ishium and the pubis. The femoral head is held in place by a thick ligament called the capital ligament or simply the "round ligament of the femoral head." Also keeping the joint in place is the upper rim of the acetabulum and the fact that the whole joint is enclosed in a fibrous capsule. The local hip muscles also help support the hip joint.

PetMassage of the hip is similar to the application to the shoulder. It too includes frictioning to warm tissues, compression, joint mobiliza-tion, stretching, positional release, still holding and scratching.

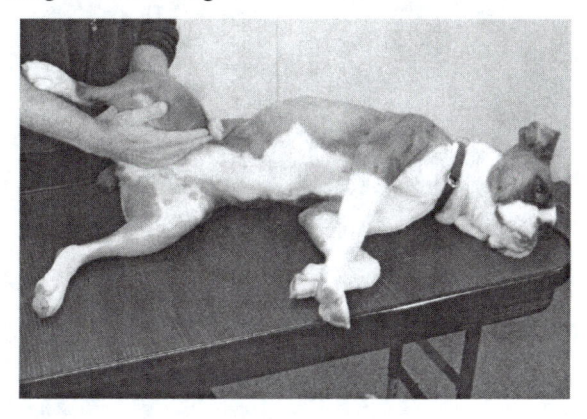

Place one hand in the groin, with palm facing out and the other over the point of the hip on the lateral aspect of the femur, upper leg bone. Press and release, gently pumping the tissues with both hands, using medium to deep pressure. Without sliding across the surface of the coat, push the skin so that it is moving across the underlying structures (bones, muscles, etc.). Continue joint mobilization, moving your hands in small circles first in one direction, then the other. Expand the movement by assisting the head of the femur into slightly larger circles, staying well within the limits of comfortable range of motion. Continue by quieting your movement, still-holding the contents of the hip joint within your hands. Breathe. With your mother hand on the point of the hip and your active hand grasping the lower leg just below the stifle, raise the leg so that it is approximately perpendicular to the standing leg. Apply positional release, observing the follow-on. When you sense that it is appropriate, guide the leg into a quarter rotation and support the full arabesque stretch to the rear.

Light scratching over the inguinal lymph node in the groin and also across the popliteal node behind the stifle, both in the direction of the heart stimulates the axillary lymph nodes, and encourages lymphatic fluid drainage. In fact, these are some of the fundamental procedures in "Lymphatic Drainage"

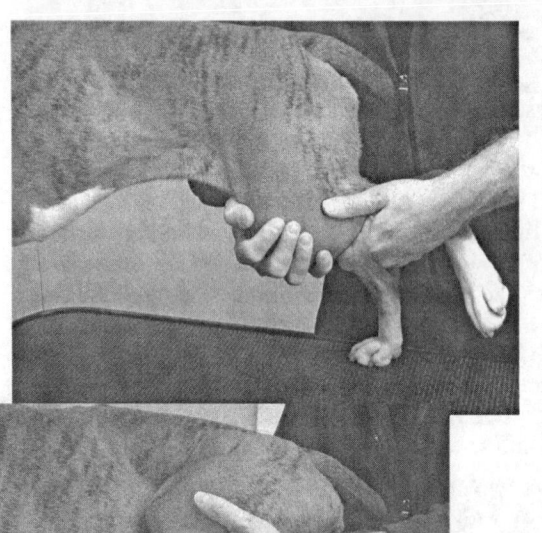

This routine increases circulation to the hip socket and leg, and increases flexibility and range of motion to the hip. Working over the inguinal lymph nodes, it supports the drainage of lymphatic fluids.

When applied gently, PetMassage is appropriate and can support normal function for most dogs with compromised hips.

When not to PetMassage

There are some situations when direct massage on the body is not the answer.

These are the contraindications, or situations when you should not provide PetMassage.

- ✓ Shock, from trauma or exposure
- ✓ Pregnant (do not work on or around the hocks)
- ✓ After breeding (do not work on or around the hocks)
- ✓ Immediately before or after eating
- ✓ If the dog has ingested poison
- ✓ Over open wounds or sores, blisters or abrasions
- ✓ Recent fractures, although gentle massage directly above and below *in the direction toward the heart* will increase blood flow, reduce calcification, and decrease healing time of recently fractured bones
- ✓ Blood pressure maintenance – do not massage abdomen
- ✓ When the supervising veterinarian feels it might interfere with his treatment program
- ✓ If dog refuses repeatedly to participate in the session
- ✓ Do not massage while food is cooking; the aromas are distracting to both of you.
- ✓ Do not percuss over the loins/kidneys, it could bruise the tissues
- ✓ Do not massage when you are focusing on other plans or activities. Your massage requires your undivided attention.
- ✓ DO NOT PRESS DIRECTLY ONTO THE SPINE. Too much pressure could cause injury.

Cancer is no longer considered a contraindication. When in doubt, provide PetMassage to the areas around the malignancy. Cancer is an imbalance of the immune system. PetMassage helps the body restore balance and homeostasis.

Precautions

Whenever possible, wash your hands before you start. Dogs have very sensitive noses and the smell of food on your hands will distract them.

There are other reasons to wash your hands whenever possible and before you start. Most hospital born, nosocomial, infections are caused by bacteria on hands. Hand washing is always a good idea.

Clean your table surfaces between clients.

When in doubt, refuse treatment. Our first rule is the same as for physicians, that is, the Hippocratic Oath "First, do no harm."

If the dog you are working on is under a veterinarian's care, always provide your work with the counsel of the practicing veterinarian. Offer to share your records of PetMassage sessions with the vet. And, maintain an open line of communication with the vets and their staff, so that you can all work together to enhance the dog's life.

There may be circumstances in which the vet may feel that PetMassage would be detrimental such as if the dog is on blood pressure medication, skin disease watch, or has had recent surgeries. An "energy" session would still be appropriate in all these cases.

It is always appropriate to provide off-the-body PetMassage therapies to sensitive areas, while not directly touching them. These include above-the-body scanning, observation, virtual stimulation, such as Healing Touch, Reiki, and color therapy.

Most physical conditions that might be labeled as diseases, in the context of PetMassage, can be described as imbalances. These are all physical situations in which the body is in discord with itself. And, as the whole intention of PetMassage is to restore balance, some aspect of PetMassage is appropriate for all of the following:

- allergies
- skin conditions
- hot spots
- auto-immune diseases
- seizures, cancer
- arthritis
- growth pains/panosteitis
- amputations
- grieving
- behavioral issues/training
- sprains
- strains
- injuries
- before and after surgeries
- for rehabilitation
- and for wellness maintenance

For your safety and for the dog's best care, the following are too dangerous for you to touch. These are serious, life threatening conditions and should be only in the care of the dog's veterinarian:

- bloat
- parasites
- mange

This chart shows the accepted contraindications for human massage. Canine PetMassage observes the same restrictions. Knowing when <u>not</u> to practice PetMassage is part of your scope of practice.

Condition	Symptoms	Possible consequences	Acceptable Interaction
Inflammatory conditions	-heat, redness, swelling, pain -sprains, strains, bursitis, synovitis, tenosynovitis, arthritis	could aggravate and worsen condition	RICE, rest, ice, compress, elevate. Sub-acute- general massage above area chronic inflammation- direct massage
Varicose veins	-veins that are enlarged and twisted due to damaged valves -can be painful	-direct pressure can cause further damage -deep draining stokes below varicosity is not advised as it may put more pressure on the valve	-spider veins ok -work around vein or move it out of the way - nutritional supplementation with Vitamin C and bioflavinoids recommended
Blood clots	-inflammation of vein -warmth, redness, -found in elderly or after trauma -may be discolored (reddish cyanotic hue)	-massage could dislodge and move clot possibly causing a heart attack or stroke	Wait for medical clearance; blood thinner medications may be necessary
Cardiac conditions	-severe high blood pressure that is unstable -arteriosclerosis	-heart/body may not tolerate increase in circulation	-work only when medicated or controlled by diet and stress reduction methods

Condition	Symptoms	Possible consequences	Acceptable Interaction
Hemophilia	- inability of the blood to coagulate -abnormal tendency to bleed -may cause swelling in joints	-usually medicated with blood thinners -deep pressure may bruise or cause tissue damage	-light pressure until you find out what the client can tolerate

Condition	Symptoms	Possible consequences	Acceptable Interaction
Diabetes	-advanced cases: loss of feeling and circulation in extremities -pitted edema: pressing into tissue leaving indentation that stays	may cause tissue damage	-circulatory strokes may still be beneficial: proceed with caution
Pregnancy	-reduced circulation in legs -possible blood clots due to hormonal changes	-miscarriage	Use Common Sense Work with physician or midwife.
Local or systemic infections	-fever -inflamed lymph nodes influenza, nephritis, hepatitis	-massage may be too stressful on the body and the immune system	-energy work -physicians approval needed
Infectious skin diseases	-bacterial infections (staph, impetigo, tuberculosis) -viral infections (herpes simplex and zoster, warts, chicken pox, -parasites (scabies, fleas, lice, ticks) -Fungal Infections (ringworm, yeast infections)	-may spread disease to yourself and other clients	-physician approval

Safety

It is important to feel and stay safe whenever working around animals. Animal handling skills are an important part of the PetMassage mix. All animals react to and complement the you they sense: your mental attitude, your physical condition, and your emotional state.

It you are friendly, the dog will be friendly. It you are fearful, the dog will be edgy, too. If you are confident, your dog will feel supported. If you are distracted, your dog has nothing to connect to, and will be distracted, too. If you are hungry, or well-fed, angry or happy, tired or well rested, nauseous, headachy or glowing with sunshine, your dog will see you as you are and respond to you according to his nature.

Dogs are social animals. In their society, there are levels of hierarchy. The top level is the dominant dog with all the privileges and responsibilities that go with power and control. The highest, the one who eats first, leads the way, such as a lead dog in a sled team, rules over the many middle management ranks, all the way to the submissive ones.

Dogs need to know how they are supposed to act They are only comfortable when they know their place in their pack's pecking order. If they sense that another member of the pack is weaker or more vulnerable, they immediately fill that power void. They take charge because that's what they are hardwired to do. If your dogs sense that you are lacking in confidence, or weaker, they will create harmony for both of you by being strong.

For the dogs in your care to feel comfortable and safe, you must develop a working understanding of animal behavior. Your communication with dogs uses the universal language of body movement and positioning and occasional sounds.

Knowing the general anatomy of the dog's body will give you an under-standing of what is happening beneath the coat. Learn how the body is constructed for movement and stability. Knowing canine physiology will give you an understanding of how the body works to heal itself and create balance and homeostasis. The more you understand about the body of the dog, the more you will see how powerful PetMassage can be in influencing health, wellness maintenance and healing.

There are a couple of elements that make PetMassage different from other approaches to animal bodywork; and more effective than the rubbing and petting your dog that you already do. In this book you are learning the theory behind the practice, the PetMassage stroking techniques, and the *way* in which it is practiced. The manner in which each touch is applied, how each touch is interpreted, and how each and every touch is integrated into the life of your dog are all imbued with PetMassage theory and philosophy.

What kind of expectations can you have by studying this book? You will learn the basic intentions behind PetMassage and the practical skills to deliver a confident, supportive PetMassage to your dogs at home and professionally.

Dog's comfort entrains with the therapist's comfort. Make sure the table height is correct for you. You may need to work on the floor with larger dogs. Support your weight with your legs when lifting dogs, helping dogs onto and off tables. You may want to invest in a ramp or steps for the dogs. Refrain from over stretching. Keep your hands in front of your shoulders. When you move, shift your weight from leg to leg.

Be careful not to cross your arms in front of you because you'll cut off your Ch'i energy as you squeeze your pectorals. The dog will respond to your reduced energy flow. Keep knees slightly bent, your back straight and vertical. Head up. Remember not to slouch or roach your back leaning over the dog. You will tire and the dog will again, respond in kind to your reduced energy flow.

Be aware of unintentional dominance movements, such as holding your arm over your dog's withers, direct prolonged eye contact, and excessive movement.

Dress for style, comfort, safety, and to complement our actions.
- Wear neat, clean, groomer's smocks, professional appearing shirt and trousers.
- Keep your nails trimmed so they cannot scratch the dog's eyes.
- Do not wear colognes, fragrances or strong essential oils.
- Do not wear any loosely hanging chains or necklaces, hoop ear rings or other jewelry that could catch or be pulled by paws or teeth.

ART AND ESSENCE OF CANINE MASSAGE
PETMASSAGE_{TM} FOR DOGS

Humane Society story

Ten times a year for the last twelve years PetMassage Foundation Workshop students, as part of their training, have been providing massage to members of the transient canine population at our local ASPCA. All of the people on staff at the Humane Society look forward to our arrival. PetMassage, they tell us, helps their dogs become more adoptable. This is one of hundreds of stories.

The dogs that are available for adoption are kenneled in large cement runs in two tiers in the rear of the ASPCA facility. In the back tier, in cage one in from the end was a small golden colored dog, shaking and cowering in the corner against the back wall. She would not make eye contact. She appeared frightfully shy and withdrawn. I entered her cage and sat cross-legged on the floor next to her without looking at her. I did not reach out to touch her.

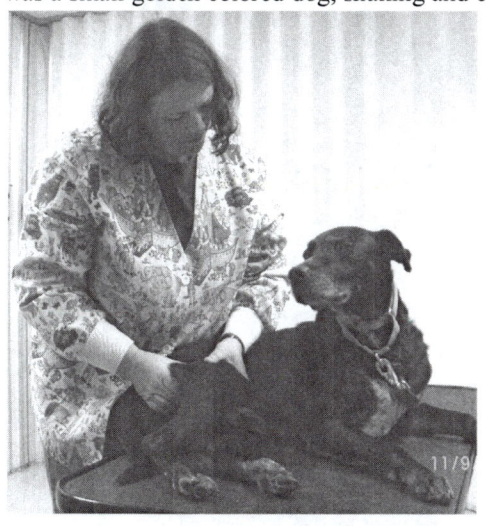

Observing my breathing I drifted into a gentle meditation. I saw myself being an oasis of calm in her world of chaos and discomfort, whatever its cause. I was making myself available for her to choose to enter my space. If she didn't, that would be okay, too. After a few minutes, she looked at me and stood up. Her head was drooped. Her tail was curled under her, between her legs. Her coat was sweaty wet. Her pendulous teats dripped onto the cement. She moved slowly toward me and lied down, resting her head against my knee. I gently stroked her head and ears. After a few minutes, I hooked a lead onto her collar, stood up, and quietly escorted her out of her cage and toward the door for a bit of outside air. As I opened the door, one of the vet techs informed me that her puppies had just been taken from her that morning. She appeared inconsolable. Of course, she was grieving the loss of her puppy family, and that was on top of the recent loss of her human family. Outside, she moved about the grounds slowly, disconsolately, disinterested in any of the scents and other distractions that so delighted the other dogs.

The students who worked with her showed compassion and patience. The massage was for her, a fifteen minute course correction in attitude and expectation. Their PetMassage was simple and non-specific. It was a means of showing this little dog that she was honored and appreciated. When the session was complete I returned her to her cage. As my role in the ASPCA field trip, I collect each of the dogs from their runs, walk them a bit outside and hand them over to a student. I noticed that when I walked by her cage retrieving or returning other dogs, our little dog began to approach the front of the cage. The last time I saw her, and this was within an hour of her massage, she was standing, smiling and wagging greeting everyone who walked near her. She was adopted that morning. If she had not had her PetMassage, she would not have been open and available to move into her new life of possibilities, potential and love.

What are we not seeing?

As we are connecting with our canine clients, we may notice a sensation of light headedness, a shift from feeling centered in our bodies, to feeling slightly out of alignment. We might feel gassy, burpy, crampy, worried, tired, lethargic. We might feel happy, giddy, excited. Our tummies might rumble and gurgle. Some messages triggers muscle contractions and the release of acids and other digestive fluids in your stomach and intestines, which cause the rumbling, grumbling sounds. *The thought, sight or smell of food also can trigger this response.* [Mayo clinic]

Our responses to real or perceived dangers spontaneously soften or tighten our skin, fascia and muscles. They alter pulse, respiration rates, blood pressure, chemistry of sweat, and production of pheromones. We may not have the abilities to smell what dogs smell. We can, with practice being present, learn to observe when our bodies respond.

You may have more awareness of the changes and shifts in your body. These are the indicators of the types of conversations that your intuitive, subconscious is having with your dog. Maintaining a vigilant presence with yourself will support the inner healing and balancing work your dog is doing. The intensity and purity of your presence, or lack of same, makes or breaks these intuitive connections.

Even if you are unaware or sense you have a block to your awareness of your bodily functions, as it were, your presence still has a powerful influence on whatever is happening in your dog's body. One of the parts of quantum theory that is becoming more and more accepted is that the act of simply observing a reaction influences the reaction. Being observant, that is, being present as a witness, supports the PetMassage healing, resting, softening and/or comforting process.

Understand the role of body language. Dogs, and animals in general, understand a basic set of behaviors. A dog from Japan knows exactly what he needs to know when a dog from France demonstrates a play bow.

Observe all of the dog's movements. Note the gross behaviors such as stretching, yawning, flattening their ears, and wagging their tails. More telling during PetMassage are the subtle reactions to touch that emanate from within the body fascia.

Assess his current state of physical and emotional health. If your dog is limping, physical health issues could be the interpretation. There could be other reasons, though, too. Your dog could have learned that if he feigns a limp, he could get more treats or attention. Your dog could have a thorn or pebble caught in the hair or in the skin between the pads of his paw. Some aspect of his body may be experiencing a trauma. Crouching, slinking, drooling excessively, and cowering, while all physical, are also certainly emotional behaviors that are affecting his physical condition, as feedback.

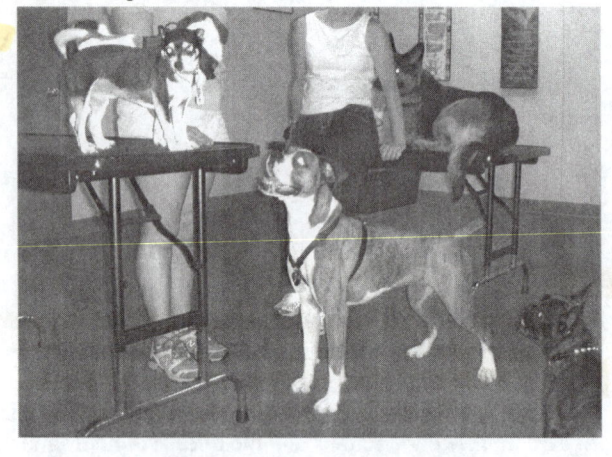

We all have lots of soul mates. Every dog you work with is your soul mate. We are all of the same earth family. We have the same mother. We have been with each other forever, in one form or another, connecting from time to time and place to place. The two of you are committed to making yourselves available to support each other's growth and development.

Each PetMassage of a dog allows you a means and the opportunity to look into your soul. The purity and unconditional love you experience, the joys, the confusions, the sense of empowerment you feel are simply your soul trains blowing their whistles.

Dogs operate using intuitive and learned reflexes. Like us, they have developed habitual ways of moving, reacting and thinking. Each of them has a personally developed matrix. A personality. Even the things dogs think about and the ways they think about them are patterned.

Their patterns determine how they are and who they are, and who they think they are. They determine HOW they think and WHAT they think about. PetMassage assists dogs in their effort to optimize their potentials and their realities.

Every movement, every sensation, every experience can be enhanced with PetMassage. Dogs' thoughts influence their physical movements. Each and every one of their bodily functions and movements has the potential to be optimized. Each can be made with greater ease.

Your PetMassage

Facilitating

We function as facilitators of the dog's natural self healing abilities. *Natural self-healing abilities* refers to the innate, unconscious and subconscious effort for an animal to move toward his/her own place of comfort...to create more safety, more balance, and homeostasis. The actual healing and rebalancing that occurs is not a conscious deliberative activity. In a supportive environment, dogs demonstrate a natural tendency toward creating a better, healthier, quality of life for themselves.

With your influence and support, your dog is moving toward his greatest good. Naturally and easily. Breathe love and contentment back into his body space. Release expectations and attachments to the outcome.

It is perfectly acceptable to express your emotions during the PetMassage. Give yourself permission to cry. Allow cleansing tears to flow. Your true voice comes from your heart and soul, not from your throat and mind. Surrender completely. Relish the moment. This is your PetMassage session, too.

As bodyworkers, we are encoded to be doers ... achievers. We expect to be able to get specific, identifiable, and measurable effects whenever we do something. We'd like proof that we are influencing situations or at the very least, that we haven't prevented good things from happening.

We want to believe that we are responsible for the changes that have happened. The big HOWEVER is we are functioning within the dog's matrix of interrelated variables. We are tapping into systems that are extremely complex. This is the biggest obstacle to making any claims in massage research studies. There are just too many variables. The lives of our dogs are a gumbo of all of their internalized responses to all of their past experiences.

When a dog presents with a misalignment or imbalance, unless they are the result of acute traumas, the internal structures are out of balance because they were in an already weakened and vulnerable condition. All genetic holding patterns, along with ones from socialization, make up the dog's body-mind, and determine how he functions. German shepherds with the potential for chronic hip dysplasia, French bulldogs with allergies, sinus and skin problems, and pit bulls with the potential for their breed-specific personalities, all are demonstrations of dogs with roots in prior lifetimes.

It would be presumptive and preposterous for us to reasonably conclude that by stimulating one part of the body, an absolutely specific change is affected in another. We cannot know for sure what the residual effects will be of the twitches and shifts we feel and on what levels of his body they are happening. Most of the releases are like dominoes, and continue their actions in the physical soft tissue that you touch., in nonlinear patterns.

The effects you observe will be the result of the natural movement of the energy in and around the dog. During a PetMassage, the choices, the layers of the onion, that are responding to your stimulation, are determined by the dog and the needs of the dog, not you.

PetMassage supports movement toward balance in what can be described as a genetically volatile environment. That PetMassage can postpone the onset of osteoarthritis and hip dysplasia shows that the releases occur within the deepest mind-body reservoirs, tempering the effects of generations of inbreeding. Clearly, spontaneous releases of holding patterns happen, even to long-standing physical and emotional conditioning behaviors. The inner awareness produced by PetMassage can bring long term calming to the stressed, hyperactive dog.

You will be continuously amazed and honored to be able to be a part of your dog's processing. One time, when you compared your dog at the beginning of the session to how he moved afterwards, you saw what you might consider a positive change. Another time, you observed no change. Both experiences, by acknowledging your presence and giving his permission to you and to himself, your dog fully participated.

Both times, he experienced *some*thing. It wasn't about you. It was about him and the choices he made while he was in hour hands. His internal shifts may have been so small that you couldn't have noticed them. Your session initiated a shift. How it manifests and what your dog does with it, is his business. A tiny course correction for a jet flying out of Chicago, determines whether it lands in Los Angeles or San Francisco.

The role of presence

One of the most obvious differences between PetMassage and standard veterinary interventions are the prolonged durations of session time, and the growth of opportunity for the development of body awareness. A complete session usually lasts between twenty and forty minutes. This could not be part of a time-efficient, cost effective medical procedure.

Although it does address the dog's acute, present-time physical condition, the PetMassage focus is on the long-term continuum of life condition. It addresses all aspects of the dog's quality of life.

PetMassage works in an open ended way. It provides a generalized experience, in which the dog's body can make non-specific, mini course corrections. Allowing the strata of intuitive connections to layer one upon another, takes time and patience. PetMassage gives dogs the time and space they need to acknowledge, shift, develop, and resolve.

When we soften our observation, we notice can more of the subtle cues that we are continuously receiving from *our* bodies; signals we often ignore. The more time we allow to actually experience our physiological responses, the better and more in-depth our feedback to the dog will be.

When we observe how our bodies are feeling and responding to our dog's reactions to our touch and presence, we get a glimpse into the inner conversation that we are having with our dogs. We become aware of the running intuitive conversation with the body-mind-spirit vessels in our hands. We touch, respond, observe, process, reorient and touch again. Each time we make contact, we do it with more understanding. We have more information, more direction, and more intention. Each session has its unique dialogue. Each dialogue evolves and deepens as it progresses.

Combining various techniques and qualities of touch, with varying depths of pressure, rates of movement, and stroke direction, PetMassage elicits emotional, memorable, and physical responses from dogs.

How can we claim this? Dogs' nervous systems react to whatever they feel. They also refer information from whatever areas that are stimulated throughout the body. The response is experiencing the memories of the emotions that are connected to the body patterns of learned behaviors.

Dogs may not be able to follow reflexology charts or understand the Five Element Theory of Traditional Chinese Medicine. They do know that their bodies feel pressure, temperature variations, and the qualities of your presence.

You're the only one who can provide your PetMassage

Only you have had your experiences. Only you have had your perceptions; your interpretations. You are the only one who can see the world and the animals in it the way you do. You are the only one who can help dogs the way you do.

No one else in the world can give the same quality of PetMassage as you.

Nobody can get the same responses from dogs.

Nobody else can have the same relationships with dogs as you.

You will never be able to give a Jonathan Rudinger PetMassage, nor would you want to. The dogs I work with have relationships that are partly based on my experiences, training, biases, and emotional state. I'll never be able to duplicate your massage. The dogs you work with will interact with whatever you bring, as you, to the table. Every relationship, every time, every PetMassage is different and unique.

The most important element that you bring to the PetMassage table is you. Within your "you," is your compassion, your love; your intention to help and support. You bring your desire to heal the wounded, mend the broken, support the abused and grieving. You would like to help all dogs live in their greatest potential; their best quality of life possible. With so many paws and whiskers all over the world, there is a lot for us to do.

Simply pay attention. Another way to do this is to not pay too much attention. Understand your role in PetMassage. You cannot heal your dog. It is impossible for you to even fathom what the real causes might be for the imbalances he presents. Your job is to facilitate your dog's natural self-healing responses.

All of your dog's inner connections and responses go completely under our radar, unnoticed.

Even if we could notice them, they'd be incomprehensible. People and dogs neither speak the same language nor think the same thoughts. Dogs and people are not the same in the ways they interpret what they see, hear, feel, smell, taste or sense. There are cultural and emotional variations. People are not even consistent in the ways we experience what we sense when we are not crossing the species barrier.

How, then, can we know what, if anything, is happening in the dog's body? One thing we do know, and this is an extension of the idea of the whole body working as an integrated unit, is that dogs experience PetMassage with the whole body, mind and spirit.

We, the practitioners, must learn to involve our entire bodies in the process, as well.

Use your body wisely, efficiently and effectively. Your posture determines if you absorb, repulse, accept, discount or ignore your dog's body responses. Your body expresses your intention. It projects your mind. Make your body posturing easy to interpret and it will enhance your synergy. The result of your combined efforts will be greater than the sum of your individual capabilities.

Release all the movements into your body, where you can observe them in a safe, comfortable context. Develop a working relationship with the earth so that you can easily and spontaneously gather its life force and ground yourself.

PetMassage Scope of practice

Scope of Practice is an important statement that both defines and limits what you do in your practice. In the process of setting our boundaries we demonstrate respect and regard for our clients and fellow professionals. This is the way to let people know what they can and cannot expect from us. It establishes credibility with your clients and your animal care colleagues.

Scope of practice
(A) PetMassage is the treatment of disorders and imbalances of the dog's body by the systematic external application of PetMassage techniques including touch, stroking, friction, vibration, percussion, kneading, stretching, positional release, compression, and joint movements within the normal physiologic range of motion; and adjunctive thereto, the external application of water, heat and cold, colored lights, and sounds.
(B) A practitioner of PetMassage shall evaluate whether the application of PetMassage is advisable. A canine massage provider may provide information or education defined by his/her training and expertise. In determining whether the application of PetMassage is advisable, a PetMassage provider shall be limited to visual inspection including observation of range of motion, and touch. The PetMassage provider shall provide services under the supervision of a licensed veterinarian including in-office administration of techniques and off-site referrals for ongoing maintenance and rehabilitation. Independent PetMassage is appropriate for dogs in the following situations: on-site sports massage, rehabilitation massage, geriatric massage, relaxation massage and palliative massage.
(C) No person shall use the words or letters "PetMassage therapist," "licensed PetMassage therapist," "P.M.T." or any other letters, words, abbreviations, or insignia, indicating or implying that the person is a licensed PetMassage therapist.
(D) All persons who hold a certificate to practice PetMassage shall prominently display that certificate in the office or place where a major

portion of the certificate holder's practice is conducted. If a certificate holder does not have a primary practice location, the certificate holder shall at all times when practicing keep the wallet certificate on the holder's person.
(E) PetMassage therapy does not include:
(1) The application of ultrasound, diathermy, and electrical neuromuscular stimulation or substantially similar modalities; and
(2) The practice of chiropractic, including the application of a high velocity-low amplitude thrusting force to any articulation of the body;
(3) Any skill that might be interpreted as the practice veterinary medicine
    (a)The diagnosis of an animal's condition.
    (b)The treatment of infectious, or contagious diseases;
    (c) The prescribing or administering of drugs; and
    (d) The performing of surgery.

It can be summarized as:
- First do no harm
- Provide only the services in which you are trained
- Do not diagnose, medically treat, or prescribe medications

The function of a mission statement

Rather than defining and limiting what you can do, a mission statement describes your goal, the purpose of the work you will be doing. It is a short formal written statement whose purpose is to guide the actions of your organization, spell out your overall goals, provide a sense of direction, and be used to keep you on track in decision-making. It provides the framework or context for your company.

Define your goals. What are the exact words you want to use to describe what you do. This is an exercise in becoming clear. It will make marketing your business much easier.

> *PetMassage Mission Statement*
> PetMassage techniques are applied with gentleness and with the permission and cooperation of the dog. We work to understand and administer to the special needs of dogs and supporting the self-healing of their special needs through the use of knowledgeable, compassionate touch, positional release of fascia, and bio-magnetic energy balancing. We do not include deep-tissue work or extremes of joint movement.

As members of a profession, we strive to always use the correct terms and language, to speak kindly of our colleagues, never diminishing their efforts and we never promise healing.

In trauma situations, remember to protect yourself from a dog that is out of control, apply CPR when you can, and get the dog to a vet.

Where do we fit in? What is your role, compared to a veterinarian's when a dog is injured and recovering? The veterinarian focuses on treating the injury, PetMassage focuses on balancing the rest of the dog that is coping and compensating from imbalances caused by the injury.

The history in the dog

PetMassage can be used to increase blood flow and decrease healing time in post-operative situations. In some cases, massage can even be an alternative to surgery. In older pets, PetMassage is an acknowledged tonic for joint afflictions and decreased range of motion. When animals are in pain or agitated, the soothing effects of PetMassage can give them the calmness necessary for healing to take place.

PetMassage channels the dog's intuitive qualities. Their activities and abilities for self preservation, include the potential for self-healing of every bone, organ, muscle, and cell in the body. Everything the dog experiences and perceives are the products of his/her long term memory.

A dog's less recent history would include how much weight your dog is carrying, how much exercise he is getting, his muscle tone and injuries he may have had.

Moving back in his archives, his influences include strongly held beliefs from his early development, his socialization, and the effects of his early nutrition. Further back, his personal history includes breed history, his genetics, and congenital issues such as his likelihood of developing hip dysplasia, cancers, allergies, and bone and skin irritations.

It has been statistically extrapolated that if dogs were randomly bred for seven generations they would revert to the original DNA patterns that were found in the feral Carolina dog, which were the similar to the DNA in prehistoric dogs [Handwerk]. Dogs carry the genetic memory of seven generations in their bodies.

What's next?
PetMassage workshops and online courses

The PetMassage Foundation Workshop
The techniques you've learned in this text prepare you for the PetMassage Foundation Workshop. This is a workshop that is offered several times each year at the PetMassage school in Toledo, Ohio. The PetMassage Foundation Workshop is an excellent beginning to your hands-on learning experience. This course is an excellent preparation for you as you become adept in PetMassage.

Learn to help your own dog and train to create your successful PetMassage business. In the Foundation PetMassage for Dogs Workshop we discuss and practice PetMassage theory and techniques, energy and body mechanics, legal issues, business and professional ethics, and marketing. Movement and breathing exercises expand your sensory and spiritual awareness and develop healthy body mechanics.

The instruction is supportive, encouraging and geared to help you to discover and develop your own personal PetMassage form.

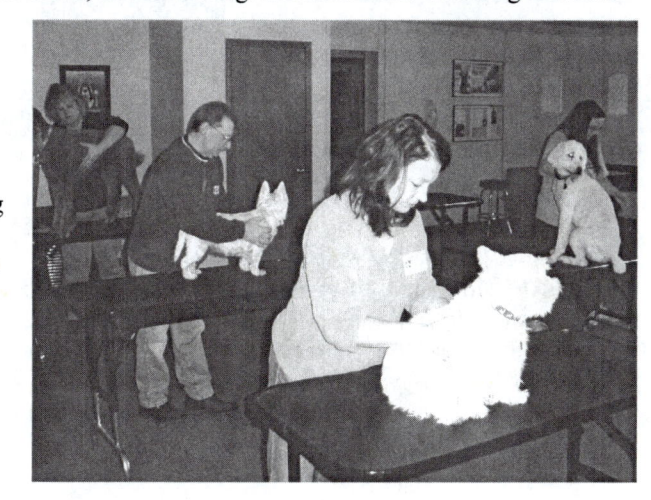

This course has been described as a personal development and enrichment class through the medium of canine bodywork.

The course includes modules on anatomy, physiology and behaviors of the dog, the affect of PetMassage on body systems, ethics and business marketing strategies. Also included is a field trip to the ASPCA to hone your skills while connecting with the dogs there in temporary residence. A Certificate of Completion is awarded for the PetMassage for Dogs Foundation Workshop after completing a take home exam and the required documentation of practice sessions.

Workshops have small classes – usually eight to twelve students. They are about 30% lecture, 60% hands-on, 10% playing with dogs and 100% growth and enjoyment. Lectures and demonstrations use models, charts, videos, other text references and the class syllabus.

The PetMassage for Dogs Foundation Workshop is accepted by RAIVE, the Registry for Alternative and Integrative Veterinary Education, for vet tech continuing education, the AMTA, American Massage Therapy Association, and the IAAMB, International Association for Animal Massage and Bodywork. It is accredited by the ABMP, the Association of Bodywork and Massage Professionals, and the NCBTMB, the National Certification Board of Therapeutic Massage and Bodywork.

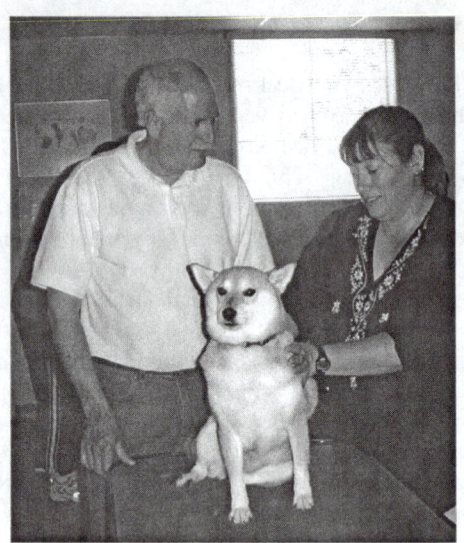

Goals of the PetMassage Foundation Workshop

- Develop an understanding of the theory, techniques, vocabulary, culture and vision of PetMassage
- Learn to understand and provide for diverse canine needs
- Learn basic dog anatomy and physiology
- Learn about various bodywork techniques
- Become aware of body mechanics for you and your K-9 clients
- Understand scope of practice, business ethics, marketing

The **Advanced PetMassage workshop** assists you further along your personal journey of your PetMassage practice. Students review, refresh, and learn essential additional skills and techniques to expand their PetMassage businesses.

The Advanced PetMassage workshop moves your practice toward massage as therapy, where your practice can be more effective when working with veterinarians and specific rehabilitation venues.

The Advanced PetMassage course provides greater depth to the Foundation workshop experience. Its training focuses on specific canine pathology, anatomy, including names, locations and actions of many bones, muscles, and fascia, and animal physiology. This is content which will help to prepare you for your test for national certification.

The Advanced PetMassage workshop also qualifies for fifty NCBTMB continuing education units for Massage Therapists.

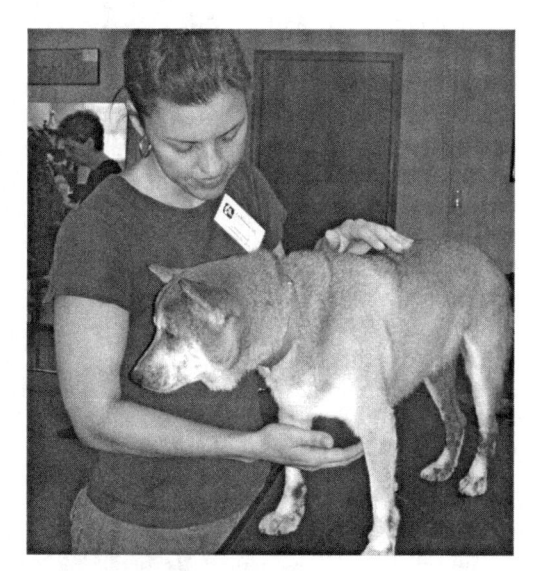

Advanced PetMassage Workshop Goals

- PetMassage students re-establish and enhance body mechanics skills and inter-species body language.
- Learn next tier of techniques
- Define business plans and goals
- Network with other like-minded colleagues
- Expand on studies of physiology and anatomy, pathology, body mechanics, ethics, TCM, and Energy practices
- To help prepare for national certification test.

Prerequisites: Completion of Foundation Course and 2 months PetMassage experience.

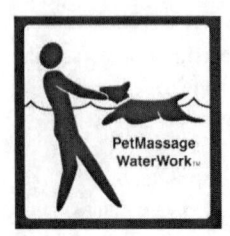

PetMassage WaterWork has a unique set of skills and body mechanics that are not part of the "dry" skill set. Part of the class is in the classroom, learning specific PetMassage aspects as applied in a water environment. The balance of the class is in the indoor heated pool, where PetMassage WaterWork techniques are learned and practiced.

Learn to understand and access water's dynamics, flexibility and therapeutic value. This workshop teaches how to move in and be moved by water expanding beyond all your land-based physical and spiritual connections with dogs. PetMassage WaterWork is growing in popularity. If you have access to a swimming pool, you can practice PetMassage WaterWork.

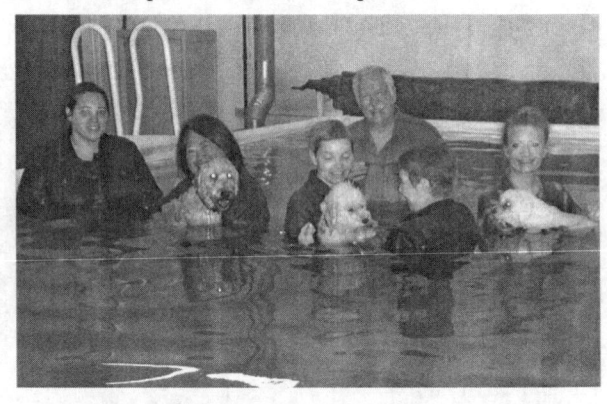

Goals of the Workshop

- ✓ Learn how effective PetMassage is for dogs in water
- ✓ Develop understanding of the theory, vocabulary and skills of applied PetMassage techniques in water.

PetMassage WaterWork is five days, 40 contact hours, and 40 NCBTMB Continuing Education Units for massage therapists.

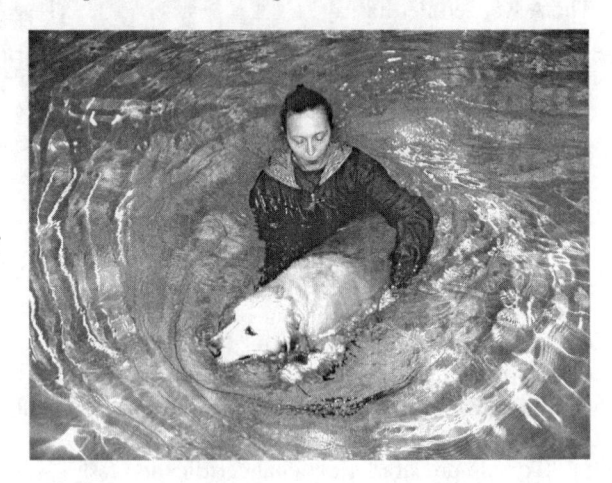

Find all the workshop schedules for PetMassage workshops and online courses at www.petmassage.com.

Online PetMassage courses

Either as separate modules of study to prepare for workshops or as independent study, PetMassage Online is constantly being updated. Discover the courses that will best enhance your practice, from Marketing your Canine Massage Business, to Canine Anatomy, to Transitions work. Find them at www.petmassage.com.

Satellite School Instructor Licensing

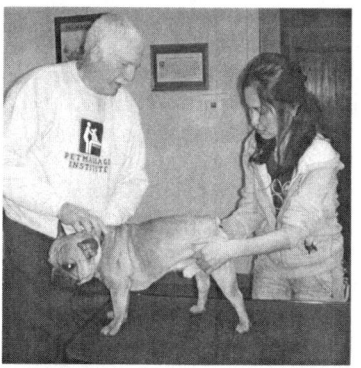

Are you a natural teacher? Would you like to generate more income? Would you like to operate a regional PetMassage~TM~ school? Would teaching PetMassage~TM~ as a career make you happy?

Until now PetMassage~TM~ has been taught solely from the facility in Toledo Ohio.

"I just wish you were closer. Then I could take your workshop!" is the refrain we've heard so often. Canine massage is fast moving into the mainstream consciousness. When workshops are offered closer to students, more students will learn PetMassage~TM~. "Build it and they will come."

Over the past fifteen years PetMassage~TM~ has built a reputation for integrity, consistency, and excellence of its training programs. PetMassage~TM~ is a recognizable trademarked brand.

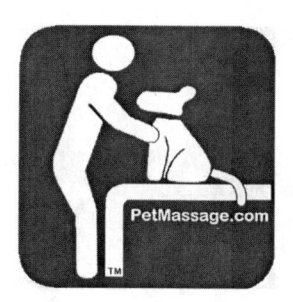

PetMassage~TM~ is on the cusp of tremendous growth. PetMassage~TM~ has been preparing for this moment. The workshops that satellite school licensed instructors teach, are the result of over 25 years of development.

More and new providers are needed to be trained to offer PetMassage~TM~. We are now training for the next generation of instructors to meet the demand for PetMassage~TM~ Providers.

The PetMassage~TM~ Foundation and Advanced level training prepare you to create your own canine massage practice. Join us. Let us guide you to take your career to the next level: a Licensed instructor at a PetMassage~TM~ Satellite School.

The vision:
PetMassage~TM~ uses its experience and standing as a pioneer and leader in the canine massage and bodywork field to provide thorough training, guidance and licensing for instructors to operate regional PetMassage~TM~ schools.

As a Licensed PetMassage~TM~ Instructor you will have a protected territory. PetMassage~TM~ affiliate Licensees will all work together as a community. Our efforts and schedules will all be coordinated to optimize and support your own and each other's success.

Instructor duties: Teaching, Mentoring, Management/Marketing, and Research. With the PetMassage$_{TM}$ Licensed Instructor credential and training, you will have increased opportunities to follow your dream and, through the work of your students, to touch the lives of many more dogs and their people in your region. You will attract students from all over your territory to attend your workshops. Your income flow will steadily increase, with workshop fees and sales of PetMassage$_{TM}$ training materials.

Train and mentor the next generation of PetMassage$_{TM}$ Providers. Teach PetMassage$_{TM}$ Foundation workshops. Teach families PetMassage$_{TM}$ techniques. Teach children. You will also teach additional non-PetMassage$_{TM}$ courses in allied non-massage disciplines, based on your uniquely personal expertise. The best way to learn is to teach. Your private canine massage clients will also reap the benefits of your career choice.

As a PetMassage$_{TM}$ Licensed Instructor, you will facilitate research studies to expand the documentation of the effects and efficacy of PetMassage$_{TM}$ using the PetMassage$_{TM}$ template. You will develop your own professional narrative publishing your books and papers through PetMassage$_{TM}$ Books.

Candidates for Licensed PetMassage$_{TM}$ Instructor must complete the two required PetMassage$_{TM}$ workshops, Foundation, and Advanced PetMassage$_{TM}$ for Dogs, and demonstrate that they can, and will, teach the PetMassage$_{TM}$ programs being faithful to PetMassage$_{TM}$ academic standards and vision.

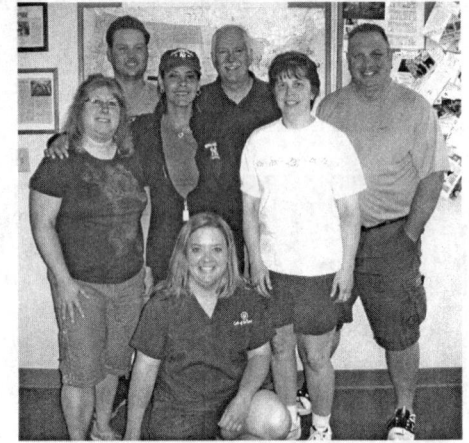

ART AND ESSENCE OF CANINE MASSAGE
PETMASSAGE™ FOR DOGS

PetMassage for kids

Kids and their families learn together to interact with their dogs safely and lovingly using our PetMassage for Kids program. This program teaches kids the valuable skills of compassionate touch, sensitivity and awareness and principles of safe dog handling.

The texts for PetMassage for Kids is the book, *Dogs Kids PetMassage*, the DVD, *PetMassage: A Kids Guide to Massaging Dogs*, and the audio CD, *PetMassage Doggie Songs for Kids*.

This is also a workshop we have developed that is being taught as part of after-school, home school, camp and scout programs. With original texts including a DVD, a book, an audio CD, and curricula, this course teaches children the basics fo canine PetMassage and safe dog handling skills.

Learn more about this valuable program on our KidZone page of www.petmassage.com. Consider teaching this amazing process to the kids in your community.

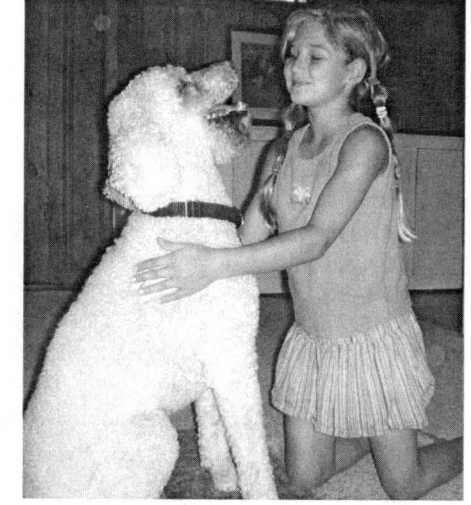

Girl Scouts. Endorsed by the Girl Scouts of America.

Visit www.petmassage.com Educator Information.

Lessons humans can learn from dogs

Here are some of the more important lessons humans can learn from dogs:

- Never pass up the opportunity to go for a joy ride.
- Allow the experience of fresh air and wind in your face to be pure ecstasy.
- When loved ones come home, always run to greet them.
- When it's in your best interest, practice obedience.

Dogs know that doing these things makes us happy

- Let others know when they have invaded your territory.
- Take naps and stretch before rising.
- Run, romp and play daily.
- Eat with gusto and enthusiasm.
- Be loyal.
- Never pretend to be something you're not.
- If what you want lies buried, dig until you find it.
- When someone is having a bad day, be silent, sit close by and nuzzle him or her gently.
- Thrive on attention and let people touch you.

From a dog's point of view, these simple tricks make for easier living:

- Avoid biting when a simple growl will do.
- On hot days drink lots of water or be under a shady tree.
- When you're happy, dance around and wag your entire body.
- Delight in the simple joy of a long walk.
- No matter how often you are scolded, don't buy into the guilt thing and pout; run right back and make friends.

Lola's story

The delightful little boxer that has been our canine model throughout the book, has a story.

Jonathan and Anastasia heard about a little female boxer that was tied up in someone's backyard. Her guardian had just been through a divorce, had a small child, a new job, a new home and no time for the rambunctious 35 pound puppy in the garage. The timing was perfect for all parties since Jonathan and Anastasia were anticipating the imminent transition of their aging boxer, Oskar and were seeking a little female to fill the void.

It was on a cold and rainy Christmas eve Jonathan and Anastasia arranged to meet Lola. By the end of a five-minute walk love was in the in the cold night air. The next day, the whole family, including Oskar, the boxer, and Jacques-a-poodle-do, their standard poodle, picked Lola up. On the way home, they all stopped for a walk in a MetroPark where old Oskar and Jacques aloof-a-do purposefully ignored the year-and-a-half old puppy. Then they came home. Within an hour, Lola was playing happily with Jacques or sitting comfortably on Oskar's back.

Oskar died about two weeks later, but not before transferring his household reign to his fellow boxer. Lola's name got enhanced to Lola Ginabrigida. Jacques-a-poodle-do: always the bridesmaid, never the bride.

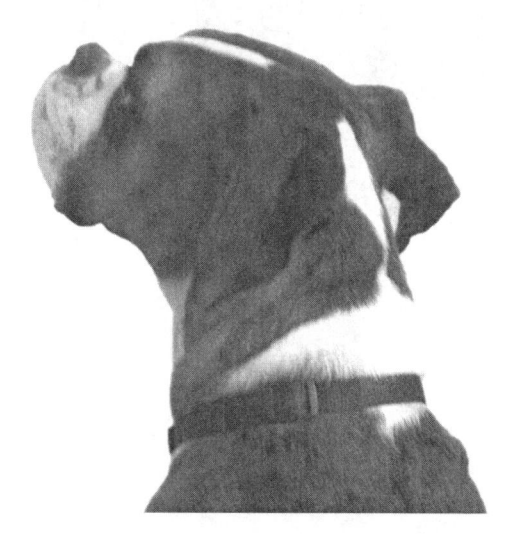

ART AND ESSENCE OF CANINE MASSAGE
PETMASSAGE™ FOR DOGS

Lola soon assumed taken Oskar's role along side Jacques as Official PetMassage Teaching Assistant in workshops. She eagerly hops up onto the table for demonstrations and discretely corrects students, during hands-on practice sessions, moving their hands with her nose and paws, and positioning herself so that they PetMassage where they are supposed to.

Lola also applies her skills and experience in her own version of human PetMassage. Jonathan and Anastasia, both human massage therapists, have a massage tables set up in their home and at the school. Whenever one of them is receiving a massage, Lola helps, whether she is asked or not. She stands up on her back legs, and with a most serious expression on her little face, places her paws on their shoulders, hip, or head and intentionally frictions, scratches, rocks, still-holds and moves her little body along with positional release follow-ons ... just like she teaches in the workshops. She knows exactly the right place to apply her skills.

This is not Lola's first book appearance. She was the star demo dog in the *Dogs Kids PetMassage*. Her caricatures, by artist Cassandra Bridinger, provide gentle humor and support to the text.

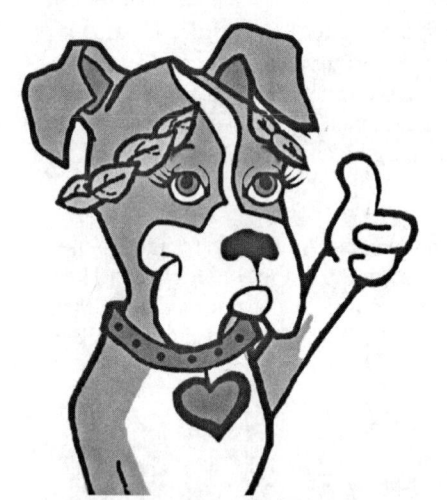

Watch Lola Ginabrigida's videos on YouTube.

Additional information for your reading enjoyment

Appendix 1 Survey

Job description for PetMassage provider

General description
1. The animal massage provider/practitioner provides massage and bodywork to animals through the use of knowledgeable and compassionate touch and manipulation of the exterior elements of the body to affect the superficial soft tissues and connective tissues for the purpose of creating physiological and psychological balance and soundness.
2. The animal massage provider/practitioner educates animals' guardians about the effects and benefits, indications and contraindications for massage and bodywork.
3. The animal massage provider/practitioner teaches and empowers animals' guardians to massage their own animals.
4. The animal massage provider/practitioner promotes profession of animal massage and bodywork through education.
5. The animal massage provider/practitioner promotes profession of animal massage and bodywork through providing services within the highest technical and ethical traditions and standards of practice.
6. The animal massage provider/practitioner promotes profession of animal massage and bodywork through membership and active participation in professional associations.
7. The animal massage provider/practitioner maintains awareness of legal responsibilities and protocols for practice.

The following defines core knowledge and skills necessary to practice animal
    Massage practice
    General knowledge massage theory
    Observation skills
    Animal Behavior
    Palpation skills

Ethics
Training
History of massage and animal massage
Business practice
Continuing education for specialization
Interactions and indications

General Knowledge
- Purpose and value of the relationship between therapist and animal
- Benefits to animal
- Benefits to animal guardian
- Massage theory
    - Contraindications for massage
    - Precautions for massage
    - Health maintenance massage
    - Relaxation massage
    - Palliative massage
- Principles and concepts of Swedish massage,
- Relaxation, attributes of, indications and applications
- Recuperation, attributes of, indications and applications
- Physiological effects of massage
- Fascia: connections and responses
- Mechanical, nervous reflex
- Psychological effects of massage
- Psycho-social effects of massage
- Mammalian Anatomy, with emphasis on specific species, canine, equine, feline
    - Skeletal system, skeleton
    - Skeletal muscles, tendons, ligaments, organs and organ attachments,
    - Cardio-vascular system
    - Respiratory system
    - Nervous system
    - Lymphatic system
    - Fascia
    - Muscles: Identification of superficial and deep muscles of the head, back, shoulders and forelimbs
    - Identification of superficial and deep muscles of the back, sides, hind limbs
- Mammalian Physiology and pathology: canine, equine, feline
- Function, maintenance, development, action and self healing of:
    - muscles, tendons and ligaments (sprain and strain), skin, hair, fascia, endocrine/hormones, bone repair
- Interrelatedness of body systems
- Pathology: common transferable (infectious) skin disorders
- Warm up and cool down, attributes of, indications and applications

Rehabilitation, role of massage as distinguished from veterinary and/or physical therapy
Kinesiology, natural movements of animals
    Action and soundness (Equine)
    Evaluation of movement
    Body mechanics: Compensation
Stress, sources of
Environmental influences
Effects of hydration, diet, exercise, massage, affection, attention, socialization
Biomechanics
Common stress areas in active (agility) dog, competition equine
Common injuries that massage can ethically address
Genetic predispositions: size, color, personality, weakness, strength, vulnerability
Application of touch to stimulate/enhance sensory awareness
Animal senses, external and internal body awareness
Healing crisis

Observation skills
    Assessment and treatment protocols
    Symmetry of muscle development
    Movement
    Gait and Tracking
    Communication: overt and subtle
    Animal body language
    Head and neck carriage, Shoulder and elbow positioning, tail carriage and caudal posturing, eye movement
    Ease and comfort of movement
    Coat: Sheen, length, odor, uniformity
    Weight, bulk and symmetry
    ROM, range of motion, flexibility or stiffness
    Legs, feet and paws: shapes, angulations and stress points
    Eyes: clarity, interest, color
    Tongue: shape, color, coating, hydration
    Nails, pads

Animal Behavior
    Basic working knowledge of psycho-social behaviors
    Predatory behavior, prey animals
    Social systems, expectations for interactions within species and with humans
        Prey, predator, leader, followers, outsiders
        Dominance/Aggression/Submission
        Hierarchy within packs, herds and species
    Role of play in socialization, Play fighting
    Fighting and power
    Calming signals

Chase response
Friendliness, dog aggression, people aggression, shyness, anxiousness, fearfulness, calmness, bonding with guardian or other members of family
Willingness to be touched by stranger/therapist
Current methodologies of psycho-social training techniques
Anxiety: spontaneous shedding of coat or skin
Emotional behavior ROE, range of emotion
    Separation anxiety, grieving, chewing, digging, barking, biting, snapping, etc.

Palpation skills
    Touch, definition and application
    Intention, holding, comforting, restraining
    Sensing animal's response to touch
    Self awareness of practitioner's intuitive response to animal's response
    Sensing empathetic releases
    Compression
    Process of acknowledging resistance and yielding to it
    Sensing resistance and adjusting stretch and compression
    Moving through resistance
    Moving with compliance
    Sensing compliance to adjusting stretch and compression
    Fundamental Swedish massage strokes
        Definitions, benefits, application
    Sensing temperature, interpreting without diagnosing
    Sensing fascia, muscle tightness, softness, stringiness, tone, atrophy
    Sensing nervous reflexes
    Sensing limitations to ROM, range of motion
    Body mechanics for safety
    Working with small animals on table and on ground
    Working with large animals
    Body language as interpreted by dogs, horses, cats: posture, balance

Ethics
    1. What the animal massage providers/practitioners do
    We work within a scope of practice (as delineated by this job description)
    Animal Massage complements and augments veterinary care with techniques and treatments not included in mainstream veterinary training and practice
    Animal massage creates an ambient environment within the animal's body and mind so that any treatment will be more effective.
    Acknowledge and work within legal limitations of massage
    Accept referrals from veterinarians, trainers, breeders and other colleagues
    Refer clients to veterinarians and other colleagues that are qualified to provide specialty services
    Maintain records of our work with clients
    Understand and abide by accepted contraindications for treatment

2. What the animal massage providers do not do
First and foremost, we do no harm
We do not claim to practice veterinary medicine
We do not state that we are healers
We do not diagnose
We do not prescribe medications
We do not perform surgery
We do not perform/provide physical therapy

3. Training
Completion of 100 – 300 contact hours of recognized hands-on training program
Development of intuition regarding natural treatments and care
Histories of human massage and animal massage

4. Business practice
Creation of safe working environment
Adherence to ethical standards of practice
Working with veterinarians as colleagues/independent contractors
Fee structures
Pro bono work
Handling referrals
Record keeping
Legal business structures
Legal practice issues
Insurance, bonding
Business plans
Promotion and marketing
Websites and internet linking
Networking
Designing office: efficiency and energy flow, Feng shui
Power of thought
Practitioner influence through emotional/physical holding patterns

Suggestions for specializing with continuing education
    Pet first aid
    Nutrition
    Exercise physiology
    Rehabilitation
    Healing Touch
    Reiki
    Aroma
    Sound
    Light and color
    Magnetic influences on the body
    Lymphatic drainage

Techniques for Swelling, neuromuscular spasms
Stress point, Trigger point
Stretching, passive, facilitated, directed
Limbic massage for behavior issues
Geriatric massage
Sensing dynamics and influence of variations in environment
Basic understanding of ch'i, Qi, Asian concept of life force
TCM Five elements
Acupressure: points, meridians
Energy levels, energetic body
Dermatomes referral areas
Yoga, Tai Chi and Chi Gung.
Active observation
Power of witnessing
Sensing subtle movements
Positional release
Myofascia release
Chakra balancing
Muscle testing, applied kinesiology
Visualization
Tui na
Distance work
Sports massage
Polarity
Cranio-sacral
Training history and current methods
Basics of homeopathy and herbs
Aromatherapy
Hydrotherapy, efficacy, benefits, role in massage
Cryotherapy, efficacy, benefits, role in massage
Breeding: standards, mixes, breed-specific behaviors and tendencies
Population, numbers of horses, cats, dogs, pet birds in US
Population, numbers of wild horses, feral cats, wild dogs in the US
Interactions and indications (Canine and equine)
Massage and individual animal care training and counseling
Massage and rescue animal populations
Massage and veterinary care
    Massage as component/complement/integrative within veterinary team
    Massage as method to relax and improve compliance of animals and their guardian prior to veterinary procedures
    Massage as preventative or alternative to surgery
    Massage as part of rehabilitation program
    Massage as alternative to allopathic care
    Massage and medications
    Massage and acute injuries

        Massage and chronic conditions
Massage and exercise
Massage and diet
Massage and hydration
Massage and hospice/palliative care
Massage and transition/death
Massage and grief support for surviving animals and guardians

Appendix 2 Fascia dynamics

Deep fascia is less extensible than superficial fascia. It is essentially avascular, but is richly innervated with sensory receptors that report the presence of pain (nociceptors); change in movement (proprioceptors); change in pressure and vibration (mechanoreceptors); change in the chemical milieu (chemo-receptors); and fluctuation in temperature (thermoreceptors). Deep fascia is able to respond to sensory input by contracting; by relaxing; or by adding, reducing, or changing its composition through the process of fascial remodeling.

Deep fascia can contract. The fight-or-flight response is an example of rapid fascial contraction. In response to a real or imagined threat to the organism, the body responds with a temporary increase in the stiffness of the fascia. Bolstered with tensioned fascia, people are able to perform extraordinary feats of strength and speed under emergency conditions. How fascia contracts is still not well understood, but appears to involve the activity of myofibroblasts. Myofibroblasts are fascial cells that are created as a response to mechanical stress. In a two step process, fibroblasts differentiate into proto-myofibroblasts that with continued mechanical stress, become differentiated myofibroblasts. Fibroblasts cannot contract, but myofibroblasts are able to contract in a smooth muscle-like manner.

The deep fascia can also relax. By monitoring changes in muscular tension, joint position, rate of movement, pressure, and vibration, mechanoreceptors in the deep fascia are capable of initiating relaxation. Deep fascia can relax rapidly in response to sudden muscular overload or rapid movements. Golgi tendon organs operate as a feedback mechanism by causing myofascial relaxation before muscle force becomes so great that tendons might be torn. Pacinian corpuscles sense changes in pressure and vibration to monitor the rate of acceleration of movement. They will initiate a sudden relaxatory response if movement happens too fast. Deep fascia can also relax slowly as some mechanoreceptors respond to changes over longer timescales. Unlike the Golgi tendon organs, Golgi receptors report joint position independent of muscle contraction. This helps the body to know where the bones are at any given moment.

Ruffini endings respond to regular stretching and to slow sustained pressure. In addition to initiating fascial relaxation, they contribute to full-body relaxation by inhibiting sympathetic activity which slows down heart rate and respiration.

When contraction persists, fascia will respond with the addition of new material. Fibroblasts secrete collagen and other proteins into the extracellular matrix where they bind to existing proteins, making the composition thicker and less extensible. Although this potentiates the tensile strength of the fascia, it can unfortunately restrict the very structures it aims to protect. The pathologies resulting from fascial restrictions range from a mild decrease in joint range of motion to severe fascial binding of muscles, nerves and blood vessels, as in compartment syndrome of the leg. However, if fascial contraction can be interrupted long enough, a reverse form of fascial remodeling occurs. The fascia will normalize its composition and tone and the extra material that was generated by prolonged contraction will be ingested by macrophages within the extracellular matrix.

Like mechanoreceptors, chemoreceptors in deep fascia also have the ability to promote fascial relaxation. We tend to think of relaxation as a good thing, however fascia needs to maintain some degree of tension. This is especially true of ligaments. To maintain joint integrity, they need to provide adequate tension between bony surfaces. If a ligament is too lax, injury becomes more likely. Certain chemicals, including hormones, can influence the composition of the ligaments. An example of this is seen in the menstrual cycle, where hormones are secreted to create changes in the uterine and pelvic floor fascia. The hormones are not site-specific, however, and chemoreceptors in other ligaments of the body can be receptive to them as well. The ligaments of the knee may be one of the areas where this happens, as a significant association between the ovulatory phase of the menstrual cycle and an increased likelihood for an anterior cruciate ligament injury has been demonstrated.

It has been suggested that manipulation of the fascia by acupuncture needles is responsible for the physical sensation of Qi flowing along meridians in the body, even though there is no physically verifiable anatomical or histological basis for the existence of acupuncture points or meridians.

Appendix 3 Healing crisis

As with all affective therapies, PetMassage initiates the "process" of self-restoration and healing. The symptoms that are presented to us may not be the behaviors that need to be addressed. For example, a limp and foreleg turn-in may be the result of a torqued shoulder which is compensating for a subluxated vertebra held out of alignment by tight muscles caused by a sore hip flexor which is the result of a swollen rear hock on the opposite rear leg. The swelling could be an allergic reaction to something in the dog's environment and the root of this reaction could be an emotional upset. You see the problem in the foreleg.

After the PetMassage, allergy-like symptoms may appear for healing because the dog's guardians requested and received a massage to help a limp! PetMassage helps your dog unpeel to his deepest layers to resolve the real issues wherever they might be.

The symptoms that you see in your dog as behaviors are often secondary to the visible effects of other underlying causes. Another way to say this is the therapeutic effects of massage affect the underlying, often deeply rooted causes that express, or show themselves as behavior called symptoms.

These unexpected responses are sometimes called a healing crisis. They surface to be acknowledged and released so that your dog can continue his life journey lightened from his dysfunctional baggage.

Each dog is an individual and will have different responses to massage depending on his/her biography. PetMassage affects your dog on superficial as well as deep levels. Massage, by its nature affects the entire body in unexpected and unpredictable ways. Its function is to assist your dog on his/her path however and wherever it goes.

The effects after a massage may include a Healing Crisis.
- Next day stiffness and soreness
- Thirst. Your dog's digestive track and metabolism have been stimulated. Hormones have been released into the blood stream. Keep fresh water available for his/her hydration.
- Limping. Muscle memory has been stimulated. Your dog may temporarily re-experience old unreleased behaviors and memories held in the fascia around "healed" injuries and traumas.
- Drowsiness and lethargy due to release of melatonin and other hormones into the bloodstream.
- Hyperactivity. Your dog may feel so good that he overexerts to possibly injuring himself. Restrict activity as necessary to prevent self injury from over activity due to release of endorphins and Cortisol into blood.
- Inattentiveness. Your dog's body has been in a process called re-education, or reprogramming. He may be confused with the new programming. It may take 24 to 48 hours for the new information to fully integrate.
- Diarrhea or Constipation. Your dog's digestive track, including the intestines, has been stimulated and may need time to rebalance.
- Urination. Your dog may require additional bladder emptying sessions.
- Seizures. Your dog's neural tube and dura matter have been stimulated. Unresolved patterns of earlier or suppressed health issues may surface due to rebalancing levels of dopamine in the body.
- Allergy, Colds. The sinuses and lungs have been stimulated opening bronchial passages in the body that were not performing optionally and releasing mucous toxins retained in the lymphatic tissues. Your dog may exhibit these symptoms for 24 to 48 hours after the massage.
- Fever. Your dog's autoimmune system is stimulated.

(Ref: Healing Crisis, <u>The Nature of Animal Healing</u>, Goldstein, Martin, DVM, pp. 163-164, Ballantine Publishing Group, 1999

> Occasionally, in cases of extreme toxicity, the body initiates its own dramatic confrontation with disease. Then even alternative remedies may be superfluous. The confrontation, when it does occur, may even seem life-threatening, but tends to produce a recovery so radical as to seem a miracle of nature. To those holistic veterinarians who recognize it as a valid process—and not all do—the phenomenon I refer to is known as the healing crisis.
>
> Of all the dramas of natural healing I've witnessed, the healing crises are most spectacular, and the most awe-inspiring. I've seen animals develop horrible rashes overnight, become paralyzed, or grow feverish enough perhaps to die, only to stage their own recoveries at the same breathtaking speed with which the crises began.

To any one unaccustomed to it, a healing crisis appears to be the final stage of a terminal disease. It's not. Generally, a pet in ill health—but not in a healing crisis—will exhibit a steady decline of energy, a continuing lack of appetite, emaciation, and persistent or gradually worsening symptoms. A healing crisis, ironically, usually follows a period of seemingly renewed health. A pet's symptoms have eased, his energy has rebounded, and his owner has concluded that all will be well. Suddenly the disease seems to reappear. Various signs of increased elimination may occur: mucousy diarrhea and darker, more concentrated urine, mucus from the nose, excessive salivation, and all manner of inflammations and flakiness of the skin. The pet's fever spikes up, perhaps as high as 106 degrees. Yet the pet, though likely in pain, seems oddly engaged by the process, as if he knows something his caretakers do not.

At that point, the animal can lose his appetite and curl up in a corner, off by himself. This is no more than an extreme case of what animals in the wild do when they isolate themselves to gather strength and get well.

If your dog's condition worsens. does not appear better or back to normal in 48 hours, or if you have questions or concerns, contact your PetMassage practitioner to reschedule for a re-stabilization PetMassage session.

References/Bibliography/Suggested Reading

Your study of PetMassage has just begun. Our greatest teachers are our clients. Listen to them. Listen to your heart. Attend as many workshops by as many people as you can. There are as many styles of animal massage as there are therapists. Even redundancy of the techniques and theories you may have already learned when taught in a new context, by a different person, to a new you, will expand your understanding.

This is a list of just some of the books and web references.

Ball, Stefan, Judy Howard, Bach Flower Remedies For Animals, Saffron Waldon, The C W Daniel Company Limited, 1999.

Beck, Mark F., Theory and Practice of Therapeutic Massage, Milady Publishers Inc., 1994.

Borcherding, Sherry, and Morreale, Marie J., The OTA's Guide to Writing SOAP Notes, Slack Incorporated, 2007.

Brennan, Barbara Ann, Hands of Light, A Guide to Healing Through the Human Energy Field, Bantam New Age Books, 1987.

Caras, Roger, A., A Dog is Listening, Summit Books, 1992.

Chaitow, Leon (1988). Soft Tissue Manipulation, Rochester, VT: Healing Arts Press. pp. 26–27.

Cunningham, James G., Textbook of Veterinary Physiology, Second Edition, W. B. Saunders Company, 1997.

Darwin, Charles, The Expression of the Emotions in Man and Animals.

Diamond, John, MD., Life Energy, N.Y. Paragon House, 1985. *Notes on the Spiritual Basis of Therapy, 7th Annual International Energy Psychology Conference.*

Felix Mann, Chinese Medicine Times, Vol. 1 Issue 4, Aug. 2006, "The Final Days of Traditional Beliefs? - Part One."

Fox, Michael W., The Healing Touch, Newmarket Press, 1981.

Goldstein, Martin, DVM, The Nature of Animal Healing, Ballantine Publishing Group, 1999.

Grandin, Temple, Animals in Translation, Using the Mysteries of Autism to Decode Animal Behavior, Harcourt, Inc, 2006.

Handwerk, Brian, Did Carolina Dogs Arrive With Ancient Americans?, for National Geographic News, March 11, 2003.

Hay, Louise, You Can Heal Your Life, Hayhouse.

Hedley, Gil. (2005). *The Integral Anatomy Series Vol. 2: Deep Fascia and Muscle.* [DVD]. Integral Anatomy Productions. http://integralanatomy.com/.

Heitz, N.; Eisenman, P.; Beck, C.; Walker, J. (1999). Hormonal Changes Throughout the Menstrual Cycle and Increased Anterior Cruciate Ligament Laxity in Females. Journal of Athletic Training (National Athletic Trainers Association) 32 (2): 144–149.

Kainer, Robert and McCracken, Thomas, Dog Anatomy A Coloring Atlas, Teton NewMedia, 2003.

Kimura M, Tohya K, Kuroiwa K, Oda H, Gorawski EC, Hua ZX, Toda S, Ohnishi M, Noguchi E,. Electron microscopical and immunohistochemical studies on the induction of "Qi" employing needling manipulation," Am J Chin Med. 1992;20(1):25-35.

Mayo Clinic, www.mayoclinic.com/health/stomach-noise/NU00189.

Millis, Darryl L., Levine, David, Taylor, Robert A., Canine Rehabilitation & Physical Therapy, Saunders, 2004.

Morell, Virginia, Animal Minds, *National Geographic Magazine*, March, 2008, http://ngm.nationalgeographic.com/2008/03/ .

Myers, Thomas, Discovery Through Dissection, *Massage & Bodywork,* January February 2010, pg.42.

Myers, Thomas W. (2002). Anatomy Trains. London, UK: Churchill Livingstone. pp. 15.

NIH Consensus Development Program (November 3-5, 1997). "Acupuncture -- Consensus Development Conference Statement". National Institutes of Health. http://consensus.nih.gov/1997/1997Acupuncture107html.htm.

Paoletti, Serge (2006). The Fasciae: Anatomy, Dysfunction & Treatment. Seattle, WA: Eastland Press. pp. 138, 147–149.

Roberts, Monty, The Man Who Listens to Horses, Random House 1997.

Rolf, Ida P. (1989). Rolfing. Rochester, VT: Healing Arts Press. pp. 38.

Rudinger, Jonathan C., Effective Pet Massage for Dogs, video, PetMassage$_{TM}$ Books, 1997, Effective Pet Massage for Dogs *Manual*, PetMassage$_{TM}$ Books, 1998, Revised 2006. Effective Pet Massage for *Older* Dogs, video, PetMassage$_{TM}$ Books, 1998, PetMassage: Energy Work With Dogs, PetMassage$_{TM}$ Books, 2004, Creating and Marketing Your Animal Massage Business, PetMassage$_{TM}$ Books, 2004. Dogs Kids PetMassage, PetMassage$_{TM}$ Books 2008., Transitions, PetMassage$_{TM}$: Energy Work for the Older and Dying Dog, PetMassage$_{TM}$ Books 2008.

Rugaas, Turid, On Talking Terms With Dogs: Calming Signals, Dogwise, 1997.

Schleip, R.; Klingler W.; Lehmann-Horn, F. (2005). Active fascial contractility: Fascia may be able to contract in a smooth muscle-like manner and thereby influence musculoskeletal dynamics, *Medical Hypotheses* (Elsevier) 65: 274.

Schleip, R. (2003). Fascial plasticity – a new neurobiological explanation: Part 1, *Journal of Bodywork and Movement Therapies* (Elsevier) 7 (1): 11–19. doi:10.1016/S1360-8592(02)00067-0.

Schleip, R.; Klingler, W.; Lehmann-Horn, F. (2005). Active fascial contractility: Fascia may be able to contract in a smooth muscle-like manner and thereby influence musculoskeletal dynamics, *Medical Hypotheses* (Elsevier) 65: 273–277doi:10.1016/j.mehy.2005.03.005.

Schleip, R. (2003), Fascial plasticity – a new neurobiological explanation: Part 2, *Journal of Bodywork and Movement Therapies (*Elsevier) 7 (2): 104–116. doi:10.1016/S1360-8592(02)00076-1.

Schoen, Allen M., DVM, Love, Miracles, and Animal Healing, Simon & Schuster, 1995.

Schürmann et al. (2005). Yearning to yawn: the neural basis of contagious yawning, *NeuroImage* 24 (4): 1260–1264.

Schwartz, Cheryl, Four Paws Five Directions, A Guide to Chinese Medicine for Cats and Dogs, Celestial Arts, 1996.

Sharir, Amnon, Milgram, Joshua and Shahar, Ron, Structural and functional anatomy of the neck musculature of the dog (*Canis familiaris*), *Journal of Anatomy*, 2006 March; 208(3): 331–351. doi: 10.1111/j.1469-7580.2006.00533.x.

Smith, Bonnie J., Canine Anatomy, Lippincott Williams & Wilkins, 1999.

Taber's Cyclopedic Medical Dictionary, Edition 16.

The Body Soul Connection,
www.thebodysoulconnection.com/EducationCenter/fight.html.

Tomasek, J.; Gabbiani, G.; Hinz, B.; Chaponnier, C.; Brown, R. (2002). Myofibroblasts and Mechanoregulation of Connective Tissue Remodelling,. *Molecular Cell Biology* (Nature Publishing Group) 3: 350–352.

VOSM, Veterinary Orthopedic & Sports Medicine Group, The View from VOSM, "Canine Medial Shoulder Instability" Fall 2008.
www.vetsportsmedicine.com/resourceCenter/documents/VOSMNwstrFallFINAL11.20.08.pdf.

Wells, Virginia, Structure and Function of the Tail in Dogs,
www.petplace.com/dogs.

Wojtys, E.; Huston, L.; Lindenfeld, T.; Hewett, T.; Greenfield M.L. (1998). Association Between the Menstrual Cycle and Anterior Cruciate Ligament Injuries in Female Athletes, *American Journal of Sports Medicine* (American Orthopaedic Society for Sports Medicine) 26: 614–619.

Glossary

Acute, disease or condition that is brief, severe, and quickly comes to a crisis.

ADLs, Activities of Daily Living, the things we normally do in daily living, including any daily activity we perform for self-care such as feeding ourselves, bathing, dressing, grooming, work, homemaking, and leisure. Health professionals routinely refer to the ability or inability to perform ADLs as a measurement of the functional status.

Agility a dog sport in which a handler directs a dog through an obstacle course in a race for both time and accuracy. Dogs run off-leash with no food or toys as incentives, and the handler can touch neither dog nor obstacles. Consequently the handler's controls are limited to voice, movement, and various body signals, requiring exceptional training of the animal and coordination of the handler.

Akashic record a term used in theosophy (and Anthroposophy) to describe a compendium of mystical knowledge encoded in a non-physical plane of existence. These records are described as containing all knowledge of human experience and the history of the cosmos. They are metaphorically described as a library; other analogues commonly found in discourse on the subject include a "universal computer" and the "Mind of God."

Animal communication any behavior on the part of one animal that has an effect on the current or future behavior of another animal.

Antioxidants a molecule capable of slowing or preventing the oxidation of other molecules.

Aroma therapy the practice of using volatile plant oils, including essential oils, for psychological and physical well-being. Essential oils, the pure *essence* of a plant, have been found to provide both psychological and physical benefits when used correctly and safely.

Arthritis an inflammation of one or more joints, which results in pain, swelling, stiffness, and limited movement. There are over 100 different types of **arthritis**.

ASPCA The American Society for the Prevention of Cruelty to Animals.

Bio-energetic We are all built from two components - biochemicals and energy. The energy of the bodies of humans and animals is known as bio-energy - the energy of life. This force surrounds every cell, providing a blueprint for the physical body and serving as a medium for the flow of information through the body. Bio-energy also extends outside of the physical body, creating low frequency electromagnetic fields around us.

Bio-magnetic energy The idea that the aura has an electro-magnetic flowing nature with colors that shift in reaction to an individual's state of mind and health has been consistent throughout history. To those who indicate an ability to see auras, the human energy body or aura is described as a luminous ovoid surrounding the physical body. Each sound, breath and heartbeat creates ripples and pulses of colorful energy in the aura. The aura is said to be the first thing one senses when two people meet.

Bloat the second leading killer of dogs, after cancer. It is frequently reported that deep-chested dogs, such as German Shepherds, Great Danes, and Dobermans are particularly at risk. Bloating of the stomach is often related to swallowed air (although food and fluid can also be present). It usually happens when there's an abnormal accumulation of air, fluid, and/or foam in the stomach ("gastric dilatation"). Stress can be a significant contributing factor also. Bloat can occur with or without volvulus (twisting). As the stomach swells, it may rotate 90° to 360°, twisting between its fixed attachments at the esophagus (food tube) and at the duodenum (the upper intestine). The twisting stomach traps air, food, and water in the stomach. The bloated stomach obstructs veins in the abdomen, leading to low blood pressure, shock, and damage to internal organs. The combined effect can quickly kill a dog.

Body language non-verbal communication, consisting of body pose, gestures, and eye movements. Humans send and interpret such signals subconsciously. It is often said that human communication consists of 93% body language and paralinguistic cues, while only 7% of communication consists of words themselves.

Borborygmus stomach growling, or rumbling, is the rumbling sound produced by the movement of gas through the intestines.

Cauda/Caudal, tail/situated in or extending toward the hind part of the body.

Centered riding a method of riding and riding instruction that is based on the idea of having the rider seated in the most effective position. It combines elements of martial arts, yoga, and Tai chi chuan with knowledge of horsemanship to create a system where the rider is centered and balanced in the saddle.

Central Nervous System, CNS, part of the nervous system that coordin-ates the activity of all parts of the bodies of bilaterian animals—that is, all multicellular animals except sponges and radially symmetric animals such as jellyfish. In vertebrates, the central nervous system is enclosed in the meninges. It contains the majority of the nervous system and consists of the brain and the spinal cord. Together with the peripheral nervous system it has a fundamental role in the control of behavior. The CNS is contained within the dorsal cavity, with the brain in the cranial cavity and the spinal cord in the spinal cavity. The brain is protected by the skull, while the spinal cord is protected by the vertebrae.

Chase reflex a response to movement.

Ch'i an active principle forming part of any living thing. It is frequently translated as "energy flow," and is often compared to Western notions of *energeia* or *élan vital* (vitalism) as well as the yogic notion of *prana*.

Chronic, long-lasting, describes an illness or medical condition that lasts over a long period and sometimes causes a long-term change in the body, repeatedly doing something or behaving compulsively

Circulatory system The circulatory system is made up of the vessels and the muscles that help and control the flow of the blood around the body. This process is called circulation. The main parts of the system are the heart, arteries, capillaries and veins.

Color therapy a vibrational healing modality. Vibrational medicine incorporates the use of Ch'i energies within living organisms such as plants, gemstones and crystals, water, sunlight, and sound. Color is a form of visible light, of electromagnetic energy. All the primary colors reflected in the rainbow carry their own unique healing properties.

Congenital diseases defects in or damage to a developing fetus. It may be the result of genetic abnormalities, the intrauterine (uterus) environment, errors of morphogenesis, or a chromosomal abnormality. The outcome of the disorder will further depend on complex interactions between the pre-natal deficit and the post-natal environment.

Contraindications a specific situation in which a drug, procedure, or surgery should NOT be used, because it may be harmful to the patient.

Cortisol a corticosteroid hormone or glucocorticoid produced by zona fasciculata of the adrenal cortex, which is a part of the adrenal gland. It is usually referred to as the "stress hormone" as it is involved in response to stress and anxiety, controlled by CRH. It increases blood pressure and blood sugar, and reduces immune responses.

Cranial, referring to the involving, or located in the skull.

Cranium, the skull.

Digestion, Digestive system, the mechanical and chemical breaking down of food into smaller components, to a form that can be absorbed, for instance, into a blood stream. Digestion is a form of catabolism; a break-down of macro food molecules to smaller ones. In mammals, food enters the mouth, being chewed by teeth, with chemical processing beginning with chemicals in the saliva from the salivary glands. Then it travels down the esophagus into the stomach, where acid both kills most contaminating microorganisms and begins mechanical break down of some food, and chemical alteration of some. After some time (typically an hour or two in humans, 4-6 hours in dogs), the results go through the small intestine, through the large intestine, and are excreted during defecation.

Distal, away form point of attachment, describes a body part situated away from a point of attachment or origin. For example, the elbow is distal to the shoulder
Dorsal, on the upper side of the body.

Effleurage a light, gliding motion over the skin that always maintains contact and directs the stroke away from the heart. This stroke is frequently used at the beginning and end of a massage treatment to invoke soothing and relaxing.

Endocrine system a system of glands, each of which secretes a type of hormone to regulate the body. The endocrine system is an information signal system much like the nervous system. Hormones regulate many functions of an organism, including mood, growth and development, tissue function, and metabolism.

Endorphins a morphine-like substance originating from within the body." They are produced by the pituitary gland and the hypothalamus in vertebrates during exercise, excitement, pain, consumption of spicy food and orgasm, and they resemble the opiates in their abilities to produce analgesia and a feeling of well-being. Endorphins work as natural pain relievers.

Epilepsy a chronic condition characterized by recurrent seizures. Canine Epilepsy is a disorder of the brain where abnormal electrical activity triggers further uncoordinated nerve transmission. This uncoordinated and haphazard nerve tissue activity scrambles messages to the muscles of your dog's body and the coordinated use of the muscles is then inhibited.

Exploration of movement the observation and *exploration* of joint and muscle *movement* patterns.

Fascia Fibrous mucous membrane covering, supporting, and separating muscles. It also unites the skin with underlying tissue. Fascia may be superficial, a nearly subcutaneous covering permitting free movement of the skin, or it may be deep, enveloping and binding muscles. Fascia is the fibrous tissue between muscle bundles or forming the sheath around muscles or other structures that support nerves and blood vessels. Deep fascia refers to fibrous tissue sheaths, containing little or no fat, that penetrate deep into the body separating major muscle groups and anchoring them to the bones. Blood vessels, nerves, and the spinal cord are all covered by fascia.

Feng Shui a complex body of knowledge that reveals how to balance the energies of any given space to assure the health and good fortune for people inhabiting it.

Five Element Theory system of five phases was used for describing interactions and relationships between phenomena. It was employed as a device in many fields of early Chinese thought, including seemingly disparate fields such as geomancy or Feng shui, astrology, traditional Chinese medicine, music, military strategy and martial arts. Wood, fire earth, metal, and water make up the five elements.

Flight or flee response also called the "fight-or-flight-or-freeze response", the "*fright*, fight or flight response", "hyperarousal" or the "acute stress response. Animals react to threats with a general discharge of the sympathetic nervous system, priming the animal for fighting or fleeing. This response was later recognized as the first stage of a general adaptation syndrome that regulates stress responses.

Flyball a dog sport in which teams of dogs race against each other from a start/finish line, over a line of hurdles, to a box that releases a tennis ball to be caught when the dog presses the spring loaded pad, then back to their handlers while carrying the ball. Flyball is run in teams of four dogs, as a relay.

Grounding using your imagination to become aware of every part of your body and where it meets the ground. Grounding strengthens our connection to the earth, so we are solidly anchored and nourished by the earth as we go about our day to day activities. Being aware of our solid connection to the earth allows us freedom to soar in our hearts and minds and spirits.

Healing Touch a relaxing, nurturing energy therapy. Gentle touch assists in balancing your physical, mental, emotional, and spiritual well-being. Healing Touch works with your dog's energy field to support your dog's natural ability to heal. It is safe for all ages and species, and works in harmony with standard medical care.

Hip dysplasia an abnormal formation of the hip socket that, in its more severe form, can eventually cause crippling lameness and painful arthritis of the joints.

IAAMB International Association of Animal Massage and Bodywork.

Infant massage a gentle and loving baby massage that has many benefits for both parents and children. The relationship between a parent and baby is enhanced and strengthened through the nurturing touch of infant massage. Parent's often find that their baby sleeps better, fusses less, and gains more weight, when massaged regularly.

Integumentary system the organ system that protects the body from damage, comprising the skin and its appendages (including hair and nails). The integumentary system has a variety of functions; it may serve to waterproof, cushion and protect the deeper tissues, excrete wastes, regulate temperature and is the attachment site for sensory receptors to detect pain, sensation, pressure and temperature. In humans the integumentary system additionally provides vitamin D synthesis. The integumentary system is the largest organ system. It distinguishes, separates, protects and informs the animal with regard to its surroundings.

Kinesiology the science of human movement. It is a discipline that focuses on Physical Activity. A kinesiological approach applies scientific based medical principles towards the analysis, preservation and enhancement of human movement in all settings and populations.

Lateral, to the side.

Limbic System or Paleomammalian brain, is a set of brain structures including the hippocampus, amygdala, anterior thalamic nuclei, and limbic cortex, which support a variety of functions including emotion, behavior, long term memory, and olfaction.

Lymphatic system a network of conduits that carry a clear fluid called lymph. It also includes the lymphoid tissue through which the lymph travels. Lymphoid tissue is found in many organs, particularly the lymph nodes, and in the lymphoid follicles associated with the digestive system such as the tonsils. The system also includes all the structures dedicated to the circulation and production of lymphocytes, which includes the spleen, thymus, bone marrow and the lymphoid tissue associated with the digestive system. The lymphatic system has three interrelated functions: it is responsible for the removal of interstitial fluid from tissues; it absorbs and transports fatty acids and fats as chyle to the circulatory system; and to Nicklas cells and it transports immune cells to and from the lymph nodes in the bone. The lymph transports antigen-resenting cells such as dendritic cells, to the lymph nodes where an immune response is stimulated. The lymph also carries lymphocytes from the efferent lymphatics exiting the lymph nodes. The lymphatic system, because of its physical proximity to many tissues of the body, is responsible for carrying cancerous cells between the various parts of the body in a process called metastasis. The intervening lymph nodes can trap the cancer cells. If they are not successful in destroying the cancer cells the nodes may become sites of secondary tumors.

Mange persistent contagious skin diseases caused by parasitic mites. These mites embed themselves either in hair follicles or skin, depending upon their type. They generally infect domestic animals, commonly dogs and other canines, but can also affect wild animals and even humans.

Medial, along the midline, medial plane, of the body.

Mission statement a formal short written statement of the purpose of a company or organization. The mission statement should guide the actions of the organization, spell out its overall goal, provide a sense of direction, and guide decision-making. It provides the framework or context within which the company's strategies are formulated.

Muscle memory Muscle memory is fashioned over time through repetition of a given suite of motor skills and the ability through brain activity to inculcate and instill it such that they become automatic.

Muscular system the anatomical system of a species that allows it to move. The muscular system in vertebrates is controlled through the nervous system, although some muscles (such as the cardiac muscle) can be completely autonomous. There are three distinct types of muscles: skeletal muscles, cardiac or heart muscles, and smooth muscles. Muscles provide strength, balance, posture, movement and heat for the body to keep warm.

Myofascial Fascia is the soft tissue component of the connective tissue that provides support and protection for most structures within the human body, including muscle. This soft tissue can become restricted due to psychogenic disease, overuse, trauma, infectious agents, or inactivity, often resulting in pain, muscle tension, and corresponding diminished blood flow.

Myofascial slings Connections of fascia that span the length and breadth of the body. There are twelve of these fascia tracts, or meridians. They connect the body dorsally and ventrally on several tracts, running medially and sagittally. They also spiral and wind so that the entire body operates as a whole.

Nervous system an organ system containing a network of specialized cells called neurons that coordinate the actions of an animal and transmit signals between different parts of its body. In most animals the nervous system consists of two parts, central and peripheral. The central nervous system contains the brain and spinal cord. The peripheral nervous system consists of sensory neurons, clusters of neurons called ganglia, and nerves connecting them to each other and to the central nervous system. These regions are all interconnected by means of complex neural pathways. The enteric nervous system, a subsystem of the peripheral nervous system, has the capacity, even when severed from the rest of the nervous system through its primary connection by the vagus nerve, to function independently in controlling the gastrointestinal system.

Orthobionomy™ a gentle, non-invasive, osteopathically-based form of body therapy which is highly effective in working with chronic stress, injuries and pains or problems associated with postural and structural imbalances. The practitioner uses gentle movements and positions of the body to facilitate the change of stress and pain patterns.

Oxytocin hormone that acts primarily as a neurotransmitter in the brain. Recent studies have begun to investigate oxytocin's role in various behaviors, including orgasm, social recognition, pair bonding, anxiety, trust, love, and maternal behaviors.

Nosocomial infections which are a result of treatment in a hospital or a healthcare service unit, but not secondary to the patient's original condition. PetMassage workers have sanitation protocol regarding uniforms, equipment sterilization, washing, and other preventative measures. Thorough hand washing and/or use of alcohol rubs by all medical personnel before and after each patient contact is one of the most effective ways to combat nosocomial infections. More careful use of anti-microbial agents, such as antibiotics, is also considered vital.

Palmar pertaining to the palm (the grasping side) of the hand.

Parasympathetic NS "rest and digest" aspect of the autonomic nervous system (ANS or visceral nervous system) which is the part of the peripheral nervous system that acts as a control system functioning largely below the level of consciousness, and controls visceral functions. The ANS affects heart rate, digestion, respiration rate, salivation, perspiration, diameter of the pupils, micturition (urination), and sexual arousal. Whereas most of its actions are involuntary, some, such as breathing, work in tandem with the conscious mind.

Petrissage massage movements with applied pressure which are deep and compress the underlying muscles. Kneading, wringing, skin rolling and pick-up-and-squeeze are the petrissage movements.

Philtrum the infranasal depression, the vertical groove in the upper lip.

Plantar the bottom surface of the calcaneus (heel bone) and extending along the sole of the foot towards the five toes.

Pheromones secreted or excreted chemical factor that triggers a social response. Pheromones are hormones capable of acting outside the body of the secreting individual to impact the behavior of the receiving individual. There are *alarm pheromones*, *food trail pheromones*, *sex pheromones*, and many others that affect behavior or physiology.

Prone position "lying face-down."

Proprioception the sense of the relative position of neighboring parts of the body. Unlike the six exteroceptive senses (sight, taste, smell, touch, hearing, and balance) by which we perceive the outside world, and interoceptive senses, by which we perceive the pain and movement of internal organs, proprioception is a third distinct sensory modality that provides feedback solely on the status of the body internally. It is the sense that indicates whether the body is moving with required effort, as well as where the various parts of the body are located in relation to each other.

Proximal, nearer the center of the body, nearer to the point of reference or to the center of the body than something else is. For example, the elbow is proximal to the hand.

Quantum mechanics a set of scientific principles describing the known behavior of energy and matter that predominate at the atomic scale. QM gets its name from the notion of quantum, and the quantum value is the Planck constant. The wave–particle duality of energy and matter at the atomic scale provides a unified view of the behavior of particles such as photons and electrons. While the notion of the photon as a quantum of light energy is commonly understood as a particle of light that has an energy value governed by the Planck constant, what is quantized for an electron is the angular momentum it can have as it is bound in an atomic orbital. When not bound to an atom, an electron's energy is no longer quantized, but it displays, like any other massy particle, a Compton wavelength. While a photon does not have mass, it does have linear momentum. The full significance of the Planck constant is expressed in physics through the abstract mathematical notion of action. Minimally interpreted, the theory describes a set of facts about the way the microscopic world impinges on the macroscopic one, how it affects our measuring instruments, described in everyday language or the language of classical mechanics.

Range of motion, ROM the measurement of the achievable distance between the flexed position and the extended position of a particular joint or muscle group. The act of attempting to increase this distance through therapeutic exercises (range-of-motion therapy—stretching from flexion to extension for physiological gain) is also sometimes called range of motion.

Rebirthing conscious-connected breathwork connecting the inhale and exhale without pause or lock in between them. It can include hyperventilation, which can aid emotional integration.

Reflexology A natural healing art based on the principle that there are reflexes in the feet, hands and ears and their referral areas within zone related areas, which correspond to every part, gland and organ of the body. Through application of pressure on these reflexes without the use of tools, crèmes or lotions, the feet being the primary area of application, reflexology relieves tension, improves circulation and helps promote the natural function of the related areas of the body.

Reiki Japanese technique for stress reduction and relaxation that also promotes healing. It is administered by "laying on hands" and is based on the idea that an unseen "life force energy" flows through us and is what causes us to be alive. If one's "life force energy" is low, then we are more likely to get sick or feel stress, and if it is high, we are more capable of being happy and healthy.

Reproductive system system of organs within an organism which work together for the purpose of reproduction. Non-living substances such as fluids, hormones, and pheromones are also important accessories to the reproductive system. The major organs of the reproductive system include the external genitalia (penis and vulva) as well as a number of internal organs including the gamete producing gonads (testicles and ovaries).

Respiratory system The respiratory system's function is to allow gas exchange through all parts of the body. The space between the alveoli and the capillaries, the anatomy or structure of the exchange system, and the precise physiological uses of the exchanged gases vary depending on organism. In humans and other mammals, for example, the anatomical features of the respiratory system include airways, lungs, and the respiratory muscles.

Scope of Practice a terminology used by state licensing boards for various professions that defines the procedures, actions, and processes that are permitted for the licensed individual. The scope of practice is limited to that which the law allows for specific education and experience, and specific demonstrated competency. Each state has laws, licensing bodies, and regulations that describe requirements for education and training, and define scope of practice.

Sensory nerves nerves that receive sensory stimuli, such as how something feels and if it is painful. They are made up of nerve fibers, called sensory fibers (mechanoreceptor fibers sense body movement and pressure placed against the body, and nociceptor fibers sense tissue injury).

Shock a life-threatening condition that occurs when the body is not getting enough blood flow. This can damage multiple organs. Shock requires immediate medical treatment and can get worse very rapidly.

Skeletal system Skeletal system is the biological system providing support in living organisms. Skin, muscle and bones allow movement. Skin - pliable covering. Muscles do actual moving. Bones give anchor to move against. The skeleton functions not only as the support for the body but also in hematopoiesis, the manufacture of blood cells that takes place in bone marrow. This is why people who have cancer of the bone marrow almost always die. It is also necessary for protection of vital organs and is needed by the muscles for movement.

Sprain an injury to ligaments that is caused by being stretched beyond their normal capacity and possibly torn.

Strains the muscle tendon unit is stretched or torn. The most common reason is the overuse and stretching of the muscle.

Supine position "lying face-up."

Swedish massage refers to a variety of techniques specifically designed to relax muscles by applying pressure to them against deeper muscles and bones, and rubbing in the same direction as the flow of blood returning to the heart.

Symbiotic relationship close and often long-term interactions between different biological species. The symbiotic relationship may be categorized as mutualistic, commensal, or parasitic in nature.

Sympathetic NS "fight or flight" aspect of the autonomic nervous system (ANS or visceral nervous system) which is the part of the peripheral nervous system that acts as a control system functioning largely below the level of consciousness, and controls visceral functions. The ANS affects heart rate, digestion, respiration rate, salivation, perspiration, diameter of the pupils, micturition (urination), and sexual arousal. Whereas most of its actions are involuntary, some, such as breathing, work in tandem with the conscious mind.

Synovial fluid viscous, non-Newtonian fluid found in the cavities of synovial joints. With its yolk-like consistency ("synovial" partially derives from *ovum*, Latin for egg), the principal role of synovial fluid is to reduce friction between the articular cartilage of synovial joints during movement.

Tai Chi Chuan (literal translation "Supreme Ultimate Fist") is an internal Chinese martial art often practiced for health reasons. It is also typically practiced for a variety of other personal reasons: its hard and soft martial art technique, demonstration competitions, and longevity.

Tapotement a specific technique used in Swedish massage. It is a rhythmic percussion, most frequently administered with the edge of the hand, a cupped hand or the tips of the fingers. The name of the stroke is taken from the French word "Tapoter", meaning to tap or to drum.

Thymus The thymus gland is located beneath the top of the sternum in the dog's chest. (The) "*thymus* activity ... involves a putting out from the heart, the spirit rising up to the Divine and going out to other people, the spirit of personal love and concern for all objects on the earth, and of course, deeper than this, an aspiration to be reunited with the Divine.

Touch Research Institute The Touch Research Institute is dedicated to studying the effects of touch therapy. The TRI has researched the effects of massage therapy at all stages of life, from newborns to senior citizens. the TRI was the first scientifically recognized institutions to publish studies that show that touch therapy has many positive effects.

Traditional Chinese Medicine, TCM, includes a range of traditional medicine practices originating in China. TCM practices include such treatments as Chinese herbal medicine, acupuncture, dietary therapy, and both Tui na and Shiatsu massage. Chi gong and Tai Chi Chuan are also closely associated with TCM. TCM claims to be rooted in meticulous observation of nature, the cosmos, and the human body, and to be thousands of years old. Major theories include those of Yin-yang, the Five Phases, the human body Meridian/Channel system, Zang Fu organ theory, six confirmations, four layers, etc.

Trigger point spots in skeletal muscle that are associated with palpable nodules in taut bands of muscle fibers. Trigger point researchers believe that palpable nodules are small contraction knots and a common cause of pain. Compression of a trigger point may elicit local tenderness, referred pain, or local twitch response. The local twitch response is not the same as a muscle spasm. This is because a muscle spasm refers to the entire muscle entirely contracting whereas the local twitch response also refers to the entire muscle but only involves a small twitch, no contraction.

Unwinding addresses the connective tissue that tightens up through activity, stress or trauma. To release this restriction the body is moved in patterns it wants, blood flow returns, health and mobility get back on track.

Urinary system: urinary system (also called excretory system or the genitourinary system) is the organ system that produces, stores, and eliminates urine. In humans it includes two kidneys, two ureters, the bladder, the urethra, and the penis in males.

Ventral, Pertaining to the front or anterior of any structure. The ventral surfaces of the body include the chest, abdomen, shins, palms, and soles.

The following are (human) massage therapy definitions [ABMP website]

Compression: spreads and applies pressure to deeper muscle tissue, forcing it to relax. Compression, or compressing the tissues against the body, induces blood flow to the areas and softens the tissues. Compression uses a rocking motion with your whole arm, pushing in and pulling back, and rolling your hands, heel to fingers. Rhythmically alternating one hand with the other enhances relaxation and softens muscle tone. Visualize a cat kneading a blanket with its claws. Throat purring is optional, although its vibration enhances softening.

Effleurage: a light, gliding motion over the skin that always maintains contact and directs the stroke towards the heart. This stroke is frequently used at the beginning and end of a massage treatment to invoke soothing and relaxing.

Fascial Techniques: This technique focuses on the body's fascia; a type of connective tissue that surrounds every muscle, bone, nerve, blood vessel and organ of the body. Massage therapists use different techniques to ease pressure in the fibrous bands of connective tissue (fascia) that encase muscles throughout the body. A breakdown of the fascial system due to trauma, posture or inflammation can create an adhesion in the fascia resulting in abnormal pressure on nerves, muscles, bones, or organs.

Frictions: These strokes are used to help break down connective tissue or adhesions, found within muscles, tendons and ligaments due to a direct injury accompanied by inflammation, like tendonitis. The therapist would use small circular motions making certain not to evoke an inflammatory response. Stretching and ice are applied to the treated tissue. Frictions are performed when tissue is in a relaxed neutral position and the thumb or fingers are used to compress the tissue over the lesion site. The pressure is increased and small back and forth movements are applied perpendicularly in the direction of the tissue fiber. No oil or lotion is used.

Heavy tapotement includes clapping or cupping, by using the concave surface of the palm, fingers and thumb held together firmly to form a cup. Light to heavy hacking is done with the ulnar border of your hand (baby finger side) and by beating with a closed full to half fist. Heavy tapotement techniques are used primarily for respiratory conditions to help loosen mucus.

Joint Mobilization Techniques: help increase range of motion. This technique only takes the joint to its limited range of motion and no further. Chiropractic joint mobilizations take the joint beyond its range of motion; which isn't in a massage therapist's scope of practice.

Light tapotement of the superficial tissue is tapping lightly with the fingertips. This type of tapotement is used to stimulate tight muscles and decrease fatigue.

Muscle Squeezing: This type of petrissage literally squeezes or compresses the muscle between the palm of the hand and the fingers. Pressure is directed slightly upwards. This should be done slowly at the beginning of treatment. Pressure will increase with each compression - within your client's pain tolerance.

Muscle stripping: This petrissage technique can be performed on a number of surfaces using the fingertips, the ulnar border of the hand (little finger side), the thumb or the elbow. The pressure is applied along the muscle fibers usually from origin of the muscle to insertion.

Myofascial Release utilizes a gentle blend of stretching and massage, to produce a healing effect upon the body tissues. Myofascial release effectively frees up fascia that may be impeding on blood vessels or nerves. This technique also increases the body's instinctive restorative powers by improving circulation and nervous system transmission. The therapist uses light to moderate traction and twisting. Results include a decrease in muscle tension, increased range of motion and reduction in pain in the soft tissue.

Myofascial Trigger Point Therapy: A trigger point is defined as a spot within a taut band of skeletal muscle, or its fascia, that's painful if compressed.

Percussive Strokes (or Tapotement): This collection of strokes tends to make brief, repetitive contact with the hand or parts of the hand. These alternating blows have a stimulating, compressive effect to the skin and tissue, thus they are great when performed pre-event or to warm up the tissues for physical activities. Tapotement or percussive strokes reflexively tone the muscles during training.

Petrissage: consists of circular manipulations with shorter strokes - such as kneading, squeezing, pushing or grasping the muscle tissue. Petrissage can be performed with one or both hands, using the hand, the fingertips, thumb, forearm or knuckles. This type of stroke usually entails an increase in pressure, deeper than effleurage, which can become even deeper by using one hand to reinforce the other. Petrissage is generally used in the middle of massage treatments, after effleurage has been performed and the tissues are relaxed and warm. The response to petrissage can be both soothing and stimulating.

Picking up or **lifting**: this petrissage technique is done using the fingers and thumbs, or with the palm of the hand. It squeezes the muscle and lifts it from the underlying tissue. Picking up begins slowly and progresses to a deep, firmer pick up.

Pulling or **Tractioning**: consists of a slow gentle pulling (or tractioning) action with the body part along its axis which causes the joint surface to slightly pull apart. This technique is performed so that muscle stability can be assessed. Pulling or tractioning is performed in successive actions which nourishes the joint and also helps to decrease muscle tone affecting the muscles, ligaments and loosens any tissue that cross the joint being manipulated.

Repetitive Muscle Stripping: Applying pressure along the entire muscle length, increasing pressure with each pass until the trigger point is no longer felt. The tenderness will then disappear. Slow repetitive muscle strippings are performed on relaxed muscles with a trigger point present.

Rocking: the massaged part is manipulated in gentle or vigorous, rhythmic movements. It ends with the body part's return to its original position. Similar to the response produced by shaking, rocking also reflexively relaxes tight muscles. Rocking is often used to treat clients with joint problems, osteoarthritis and tight muscles.

Shaking: increases range of motion in a joint. It can be performed at the beginning, middle or end of a treatment, on tight muscles. Shaking affects the sensory nerves in the muscles and joints that reflexively relaxes the client and reduces the muscle tightness within. The action is done by grasping either the muscle belly, for direct shakings, or the limb furthest away from the body, for indirect shakings. The tissue is then moved back and forth at an even rhythm - from gentle to vigorous.

Skin Rolling: This petrissage technique lifts the skin between the thumb and fingers and is gently rolls over the area, very slowly. Skin rolling allows a release in the superficial restrictions between the skin and underlying tissue. It may be necessary to repeat rolling a few times over the same area in order to release any long term adhesions.

Stroking: This is one of the lightest petrissage techniques. The skin alone is stroked, so that the underlying tissue is not directly affected. Any part of the hand or fingers can be used to perform this rhythmic stroke. Stroking produces a stimulating effect with its multidirectional strokes, random rhythm and rate. Stroking is commonly used to end a treatment.

It can be a soothing stroke if the client wishes to relax and stimulating if the client wishes to be alert.

Wringing: is a rhythmic picking up the tissue. Wringing fills the hand and tosses the tissue back and forth between in opposition. Your hands will conform to the tissue and the depth of the pressure will increase when tissue is lifted and torqued. The pressure eases when the hands return to their original starting position. A type of petrissage.

Vibrations: are applied lightly to the surface of the skin and vibrated or moved at a rapid rate. Vibrations are performed statically (in one place) or running (along the skin's surface). The trembling action of the hands and fingers transfers to the client rendering various results. For instance, when vibration is done briskly it becomes stimulating, but when it is performed gently it helps to relax and reduce any tension. This is another type of petrissage.

Anatomical Terms: Directions, Locations and Shapes

Dorsal- Upper side or top of dog's body

Ventral- Underside or bottom of dog's body

Superior- Above

Supra- (abbreviation) above

Inferior- Below

Sub- (abbreviation) under

Proximal- Closer to midline of body

Distal- Further away from midline of body

Midline- Center of body i.e. spine is midline

Sagittal plane- Vertical plane through longitudinal axis of the trunk dividing the body into right and left halves

Lateral- On the outside (of the limb)

Medial- Toward the middle, on the inside of the limb

Contralateral- Corner to opposite corner, as in upper right and lower left

Ipsilateral- being on or affecting the same side of body

Inguinal- Refers to the groin

Lingual- Refers to the tongue

Crest- Ridge or elongated prominence

Protuberance- Bulge, a part that is prominent above the surface, like a knob

Rostral- Refers to beak or snout of animal

Caudal- Refers to tail, rear

Cranial- Refers to head, front of body

Abduction- Bringing limb toward medial line

Adduction- Pushing limb away from medial line

Index

Abduction 102, 106
Acetabulum 219
Achilles tendon 89
Active hand 100, 134-7, 161
Acute 107
Adhesions 112, 114
ADLs, Activities of Daily Living 23
Adduction 102, 106
Adrenaline 171
Agility 21, 145
Agonist 102
Air flow 170-1
Akashic record 19
Alpha state 144
Amputated limbs 87
Anatomy 102, 226
Animal communication 14
Antagonist 102
Antioxidants 50
Anxious dog 44
Aromas 13, 40, 170-2
Arrector pili muscle 45
Arterial rhythm 153
Arthritis 67, 104
Articular cartilage 101
Articulation 101
ASPCA 227-28
Assessment stroking 40, 86, 86-91, 182-3
Attachment sites 65
Axillary/axilla lymph node 154, 218

Balance 104, 131, 209
Ball and socket joint 102, 219
Belly to middle back 74
Benefits 207
Bio-energetic currents 50
Bio-magnetic energy field 59
Bio rhythms 68
BIRP 204
Bloat 223
Blowing coat 44
Body breath 139-40, 142
Body chemistry 46
Body language 26, 40, 43, 230
Body Mechanics 79, 163, 168, 173
Body systems 153
Body wisdom 132
Borborygmus 173
Bowel movements 93
Breath, Breathe, breathing 63, 103, 113, 135, 150, 155, 161
Breed characteristics 130
Breed memories 57, 130
Buddha smile 64, 164

Cancer 221
Candles 170
Capital ligament 219
Capsular ligaments 101
Cardiovascular circulation 82
Carpets 166-7
Carolina dog 243
Casey, Edgar 19
Cauda, caudal 72, 106
Cellular memory 129
Centered riding 15
Central Nervous System 71, 74, 125
Cerebral Spinal Fluid (CSF) 157
Cervical vertebrae 215
Chase reflex 50, 60
Chi 81, 156-7, 226
Chiropractics 103
Chronic, 107
Circulatory system 154, 157
Clasped hands 95, 187
Clearing energy 161
Closing ritual 159-61
Coat 147
Coccyx 72
Compensation 128
Compression 40, 49, 97, 99, 132, 139, 185, 188, 190-1

Congenital diseases 57
Connect the dots 159, 196
Connections 84
Conscious-connected breathwork 25
Constipation 118
Continued movement 139
Contraindications 221
Cool areas 66
Cool down 211
Cortisol 45
Course corrections 129, 235
Cramps 147
Cranial 106
Cross-fiber 83
Cross skin-rolling 111, 186
Crufts Show 22
Cultural memories 128
Cupping 120-21, 187

Deep work 97
Defining a dog 130
Detroit Kennel Club 21
Diagnose 104, 240-1
Diaphragm 95, 155
Digestion 93
Digestive system 155, 157
Disclaimer 206
Disconnecting 150, 198
Distal 106
Distractions 144, 170
DNA 243
Documentation 203
Dominance Movements 163, 215, 226
Do no harm 105, 172, 222, 241
Dorsal 106
Dress 226
Dressage 15
Dysplasia 107, 178

Ears 87
Earth Ch'i 81
Echinacea 172
Effleurage 40, 78, 79
Elimination 201
Ellipsoidal joint 102
Emotional response 129
Empathetic participation 132, 142
Endocrine system 156-7
Endorphins 50

Epilepsy 170
Equine Affaire, The 20
Erect stance 43
Esophagus 73
Essential oil 170, 172
Expectations 131, 226, 234-5
Expectoration 120
Expansion 132, 136, 139
Exploration of movement 134, 136-7, 216
Extension 102, 106
Extensors 145

Facilitating 234, 238
Fascia 101, 139, 145, 151-2, 261-262
Fascia meridians 68
Fatty pockets 66
Feng Shui 171, 173
Fibrous joint capsule 101
Fight or flight, fight or flee response 45, 171
Finger flicking 118
Fingernails 95
Fingertip compression 185
Fingertip tapping 116
Flexion 102, 106
Flexors 15
Floor 165-7
Florescent lights 137, 170
Flyball 21, 145
Follow-on 109, 132, 140-41
Footwork 114
Friction, frictioning 40, 112, 114, 184, 188

Gasp 128
Geriatric PetMassage 93, 208
Gliding joint 102
Grieving 222
Grooming table 166
Ground, Grounding 160, 173, 197

Hair follicles 40
Hair patterns 67
Hand position 53, 76
Head postures 215
Healing Crisis 130, 263-265
Healing Touch 222
Heart 73
Heavy rain drops 116-17
Hinge joint 102
Hip 219-20

Hip dysplasia 67, 178
Hippocratic Oath 222
Hippocrates 33
History 243
Hocks 103
Holding patterns 128-30
Holding your breath 150
Holograms 136
Hot spots 222
Hydration 201
Hydration 198

IAAMB, Int'l Assn of Animal Massage and Bodywork 29
Ilium 72
Imaging 202
Immune system 154, 172
Infant massage 25
Inflammation 66
Inguinal lymph node 154, 220
Inner dialogue 129, 144
Intake form 205
Integration shake 21, 162, 200
Integumentary system 153, 157
Intercostal muscles 95
internal visualization 142
Internalizing releases 142
Insertions 66
Ischium 72
Ischial tuberosity 89

Job Description 30, 254-260
Joints 145
Joint capsule 66, 138
Joint mobilization 41, 100, 112, 124, 139, 185, 188, 213
Joint stability 102
Joints, swollen 66
Join-up 44
Jostling 124
Judgments 131

Kegels 109
Kids PetMassage program 248
Kinesiology 136
Kidneys 117
Kneading 40, 108, 110
Knuckles 83, 112
Krupa, Gene 61

Lateral 106

Lavender 172
Ligaments 101
Limbic System 74, 125
Light 170
Light refracting 45
Ling, Per Henrik 33
Liver 95
Lola 250-1
Lumps 66
Lungs 73
Lymphatic system 93, 153-4, 157
Lymph drainage 93, 216, 220

Mange 223
Massage table 166, 173
Medial 88, 106
Memories 139
Metabolic waste 147
Mission Statement 242
Morningstar Jim, 25
Mother Earth 160
Mother hand 100, 134-7, 161, 217
Mouthing 67
Movement 101
Mucus 118
Muscle knots 83
Muscle memory 36, 109, 139
Muscle Squeezing 113
Muscle tightness 65
Muscular system 154, 157
Music 14, 170, 172
Myofascial release 133
Myofascial slings 151

Narrative notes 204
Nature sounds 172
Neck 214-16
Neolithic wall paintings 34
Nerve plexuses 74
Nervous system 155
Non-compliant 45
Nosocomial 222

Observation 132, 179, 199
Obese dogs 215
Online PetMassage courses 247
Open hand percussing 119
Origins 65
Orr, Leonard 25

Orthobionomy™ 28
Oxytocin 45

Palms 61, 72, 95, 114, 118, 126
Palpation 60
Parasites 223
Pare, Ambroise 33
Peristalsis 118
Paw 145
Pelvic girdle 72
Perception 129
Percussive strokes 116
Pericardium 73
Peripheral nerves 40
Permission 40, 42, 47, 173, 179, 234
Personal space 40, 42
Petrissage 40, 108
Pheromones 161
Philtrum 87, 88
Phlegm 120
Physical therapy 103
Picking up 108, 111
PIRP 204
Place of comfort 134
Plantar 89
Popliteal lymph node 154, 220
Positional release 103, 109. 124, 133-46, 185, 189, 190
Postures 43, 128
Precautions 222
Prescapular lymph node 153
Presence 236
Pressure, Deep 57
Pressure, Medium 56
Proprioception 125
Proximal 106
Pubis 72
Pulling 104
Pupils 43
Push back 135-6, 138, 140

Qi 156-7
Quantum mechanics 60, 132

Raised hackles 44
Range of emotion, ROE 124
Range of motion, ROM 100, 124, 220
Rates of movement 94
Reactive movement massage 131
Re-assessment strokes 192

295

Rebirthing 25, 28
Recoil 137, 140
Reflexive responses 131
Regroup 173
Rehabilitation 222
Reiki 222
Repetitive scratching 94
Repetitive stroking 94
Relationships 132
Releases 142, 201
Reproductive system 156-7
Resistance 173-4
Resolution 132
Respiratory conditions 118
Respiratory system 155, 157
Retraction 132
Rocking 125-27, 185, 187, 191
Rolling 97
Rostral 106
Rotation 102, 106
Rule of Halves 73

Sacrum 72
Saddle joint 102
Safety 225
Scope of practice 103, 104, 223, 240-41
Scratch, scratching 40, 92-3, 186, 189, 218, 220
Seizures 170
Sense of smell 171
Sensory nerves 124
Shaking 124-25
Shock 221
Shoulder 217-18
Side-lying 126
Skeletal muscles 101
Skeletal system 154, 157
Skin 145
Skin bracelets 53
Skin rolling 41, 110-12, 138-9, 162, 184, 186
Skin rolling with a twist 112
Slapping 119
Snapping fingers 112
SOAP 204
Softened coat 44
Somatic nervous system, 155
Sound 40
Spleen 95, 154
Sports massage 103, 209-11
Sprain 66, 107, 222

Stagnant air 171
Still-holding 51, 68, 99, 133, 194
Stillness 51, 60
Still-print 51, 52, 55
Strain 66, 107, 222
Stress hormones 171
Stretching 132, 137-9, 147-9, 209
String of pearls 80
Stroke, stroking 40, 78, 80-3
Stroke, Directions 82
Subconscious 129
Submandibular lymph node 153
Submissive dogs 43, 212
Supine120, 149
Sweat wrap 99
Sweaty palms 45
Swedish massage 35
Swelling 66
Symbiotic relationship 34
Symptom 131
Synergist 102, 147
Synergist functions 153
Synovial fluid 66, 101, 102
Synovial joints 101, 102
Synovial membrane 101

Table 166, 173
Table Manners 169
T'ai Ch'i Chuan 25, 80
T'ai Ch'i exercise 64
Tail 87, 191, 212-14
Tapotement 116, 120
Tapping 184, 187
Tender spots 67
Tendons 101
Thanking 198
Thumb 53
Thumb walk 184
Thymus 123
Thymus thump 122, 198
Touch 40, 49, 50
Touch, Light 55
Touch-print 52, 86
Touch Research Institute 49
Traction, Tractioning 103, 133, 137
Transitions 59
Tribe 28
Trigger points 83

297

Ulnar border 118
Unwinding 133, 134, 135, 143
Urinary system 156-7

Vector, vectoring 68, 69, 76, 137, 180, 194
Venous blood flow 93
Ventral 90, 106
Visualize, visualization 68, 80, 96, 102, 143, 161, 202

Warm areas 66
Warm up 209-10
Warts 66
WaterWork 247
Westminster Kennel Club 22
Winding 137-8
Witnessing 139, 143
Workshops 244-7
Wrist 53

Xyphoid process 74

Yawn reflex 149

More fine PetMassage™ Books, DVDs, and CDs

PetMassage Energy Work With Dogs

Accessing The Magnificent Body Language & Body Wisdom of the Dog through Acupressure, Chakra Balancing & Positional Release

See review in American *Holistic Veterinary Medical Association* July – September 2006

Your PetMassage and your canine clients will be more profound, focused and transformative. **PetMassage Energy Work** will add a new dimension to your PetMassage.

PetMassage Energy Work With Dogs incorporates the use of energy in your PetMassage work. Learn to use and enhance the effects of touch, positional release, acupressure, chakra work and communication fundamentals in your practice.

PetMassage Energy Work with Dogs, 326 pages, with photographs, charts, exercises, index and glossary. $34.95

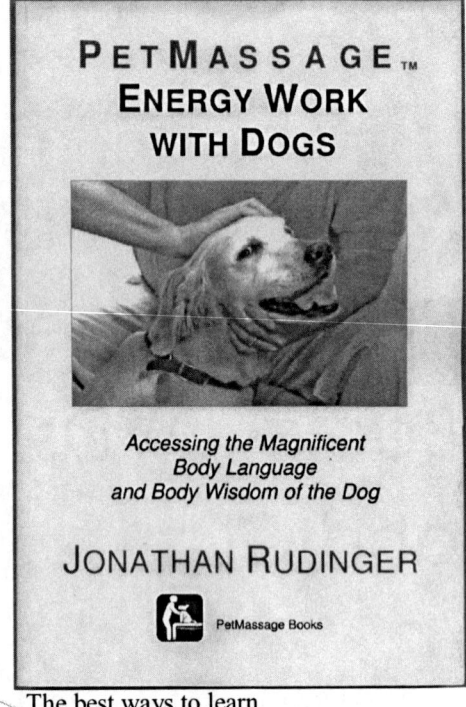

The best ways to learn **PetMassage Energy Work** are to read it, listen to it, and practice it.

Learn while driving around with the set of 5 Audio CD's 5 hours, 52 minutes.

PetMassage Energy Work With Dogs book $34.95

PetMassage Energy Work With Dogs 5-CD set $44.95

TRANSITIONS PetMassage Energy Work for the Aging & Dying Dog celebrates life ... and death. This is a book of hope and love that will comfort you during the difficult times of impending loss.

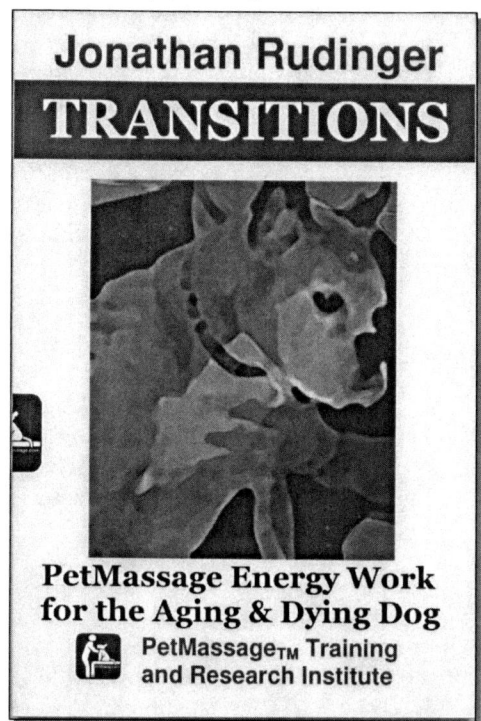

TRANSITIONS teaches ways to be empowered during the last few months of your dog's life. It chronicles the story of the last days of Oskar the boxer, and the powerful last PetMassage session, author Jonathan Rudinger, shared with his cherished canine PetMassage teaching assistant. This is a beautiful guide in the use of touch and intention for sharing a loving goodbye.

TRANSITIONS PetMassage Energy Work for the Aging & Dying Dog only $20.

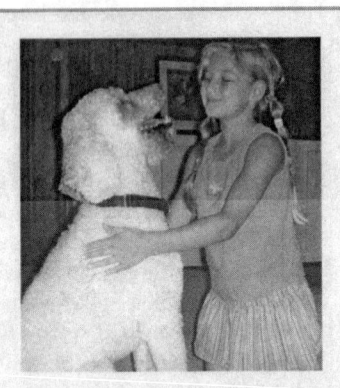

ART AND ESSENCE OF CANINE MASSAGE
PETMASSAGE TM FOR DOGS

PetMassage_{TM} for the Family Dog

PetMassage_{TM} for the Family Dog expands on the massage you do intuitively with the skills and theory of professional canine massage therapy. PetMassage is easy to learn and fun to give. And your dogs, well, this is great return on their investment of unconditional love they give you!

Follow PetMassage School star teaching assistant, Standard Poodle, Jacques a Poodle-Do, with his person, Jonathan Rudinger, as you learn to give your dog a confident, nurturing canine PetMassage.

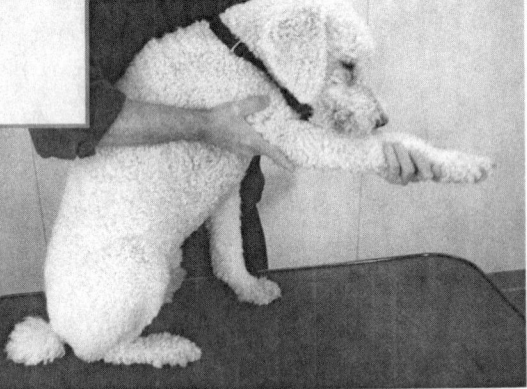

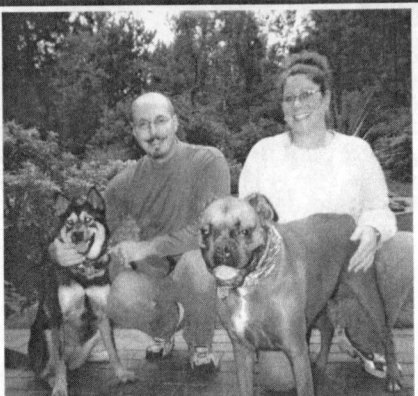

Topics covered:
- ✓ benefits of massage
- ✓ techniques & sequences
- ✓ older (Geriatric) dog massage
- ✓ therapies for upper spine and back, respiratory enhancement, hips
- ✓ use of additional methods of acupressure, exploration of movement, respiratory enhancement and visualization.

164 pages, incl. 159 photos, index, & reading list. $29.95 + $7.00. S/H

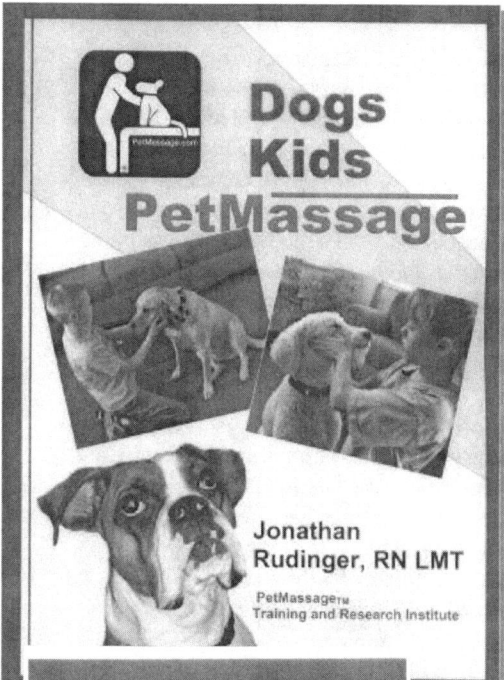

PetMassage for Kids

The therapeutic power of touch along with the enjoyment and value of PetMassage join with the natural connection children have with their dogs. Learning and practicing PetMassage is more than just petting dogs!

This program teaches kids the valuable skills of compassionate touch, sensitivity and awareness and principles of safe dog handling.

This is the perfect (educational) gift for every child who loves dogs.

PetMassage for Kids is a 3-part set **Dogs Kids PetMassage,** book, **PetMassage: A Kids Guide to Massaging Dogs,** the 60-minute DVD, **PetMassage Doggie Songs for Kids** audio CD.

PetMassage for Kids is the study material for families, after school, home school, camp and scout programs.

Dogs Kids PetMassage book $16.95.

PetMassage: A Kids Guide to Massaging Dogs, DVD $17.95 **PetMassage Doggie Songs for Kids** Audio CD $12.95

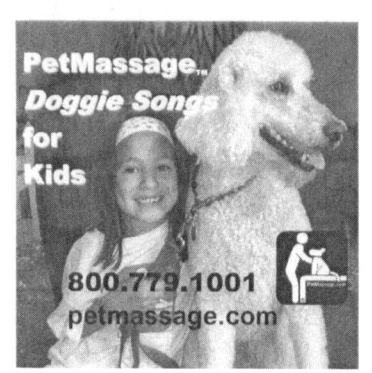

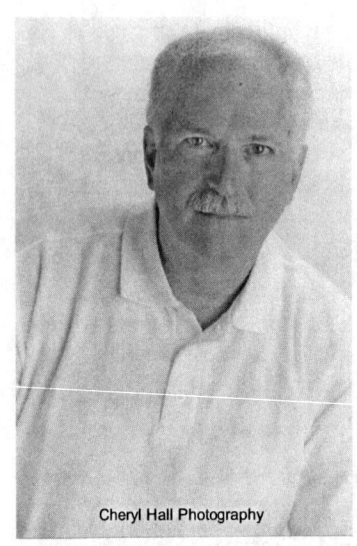

About the author

Jonathan Rudinger, Registered Nurse and Licensed Massage Therapist, has been instrumental in the development and acceptance of animal massage since the mid-1990's. He has facilitated over 300 weeklong canine PetMassage training workshops at the PetMassage school in Toledo, Ohio. His home study courses have provided instruction for thousands of dog caregivers all over the world. His on-line and independent study courses are tailored to meet the needs of his students.

An authority on massage for dogs, Jonathan has been interviewed on National Public Radio, and many major radio and national television and cable networks. He has been featured in *Whole Dog Journal, Dog Fancy Magazine, Natural Dog Magazine, Cosmopolitan, Glamour, AARP Magazine, Massage Magazine, Animal Wellness Magazine, Massage Today and Massage Therapy Journal.* Jonathan is a featured presenter at H.H. Backer Pet Industry Trade Shows.

Jonathan is the founder and president of the International Association of Animal Massage and Bodywork, www.iaamb.org.

Jonathan and Anastasia, his partner in life and business, teach, massage, live and love with their two dogs, Lola Ginabrigida and Jacques-a-poodle-do, in Toledo, Ohio.